ROUTLEDGE LIBRARY EDITIONS: NURSE EDUCATION AND NURSING CARE

Volume 11

SOCIAL SKILLS TRAINING AND PSYCHIATRIC NURSING

SOCIAL SKILLS TRAINING AND PSYCHIATRIC NURSING

OWEN HARGIE
AND
PATRICK McCARTAN

Routledge
Taylor & Francis Group

LONDON AND NEW YORK

First published in 1986 by Croom Helm Ltd.

This edition first published in 2026
by Routledge
4 Park Square, Milton Park, Abingdon, Oxon OX14 4RN

and by Routledge
605 Third Avenue, New York, NY 10158

Routledge is an imprint of the Taylor & Francis Group, an informa business

British Library Cataloguing in Publication Data
A catalogue record for this book is available from the British Library

ISBN: 978-1-041-11658-5 (Set)
ISBN: 978-1-041-10324-0 (Volume 11) (hbk)
ISBN: 978-1-041-10337-0 (Volume 11) (pbk)
ISBN: 978-1-003-65453-7 (Volume 11) (ebk)

DOI: 10.4324/9781003654537

Publisher's Note
The publisher has gone to great lengths to ensure the quality of this reprint but points out that some imperfections in the original copies may be apparent.

Disclaimer
The publisher has made every effort to trace copyright holders and would welcome correspondence from those they have been unable to trace.

Social Skills Training and Psychiatric Nursing

OWEN HARGIE and PATRICK McCARTAN

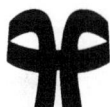

CROOM HELM
London • Sydney • Dover, New Hampshire

Croom Helm Ltd, Provident House, Burrell Row,
Beckenham, Kent BR3 1AT
Croom Helm Australia Pty Ltd, Suite 4, 6th Floor,
64-76 Kippax Street, Surry Hills, NSW 2010 Australia

British Library Cataloguing in Publication Data

Hargie, Owen
Social skills training and psychiatric
nursing.
1. Mentally ill — Rehabilitation
2. Social skills — study and teaching.
I. Title.   II. McCartan, Patrick
362.2'1   RC489.S63

ISBN 0-7099-3749-0

Croom Helm, 51 Washington Street, Dover,
New Hampshire 03820, USA

Library of Congress Cataloging-in-Publication Data

Hargie, Owen.
Social skills and psychiatric nursing.

Bibliography: p.
Includes index.
1. Social skills—therapeutic use. 2. Psychiatric
nursing. 3. Nurse and patient. I. McCartan, P.J.
(Patrick John) II. Title. (DNLM: 1. Adaptation,
psychological—nurses' instruction. 2. Nurse-patient
relations. 3. Psychiatric nursing. 4. Social behavior—
nurses' instruction. WY 160 H279S)
RC489.S63H37   1986   610.73'68   86-6325
ISBN 0-7099-3749-0 (pbk.)

Typeset in 10pt Times by Leaper & Gard Ltd, Bristol, England
Printed and bound in Great Britain by Mackays of Chatham Ltd, Kent

CONTENTS

For: Patricia, Ethel
Carmel, Ciara, Eimear, Margaret

'Mental illness often fundamentally affects social adjustment, even after the primary symptoms of the illness have been treated. If the patient is to resume his place in a busy, competitive society, he will need help in regaining social skills which in the ordinary person are taken for granted.'

Better Services for the Mentally Ill. (HMSO, 1975)

1 INTRODUCTION

During the past two decades interest in the field of social interaction has developed rapidly. In particular, attention has been devoted to three main aspects: firstly, the actual repertoire of social behaviour displayed by individuals; secondly, why some people are better social interactors than others; and thirdly, attempts to introduce training programmes designed to improve the communicative ability of individuals. All three of these aspects are important within psychiatry, in that we need to understand why some patients may be less socially skilled, we should be concerned with the development of methods to help such patients improve their social skills, and, in order to do so, we need to be able to identify exactly in which social behaviours these patients demonstrate deficits.

Ellis and Whittington (1981) have identified three main contexts within which programmes of social skills training (SST) have been initiated:

(1) Developmental. Here the concern is with the development of appropriate social behaviour in young children and SST programmes have been implemented both for children thought to be at risk of mental illness or behaviour disorder, and for normal children

(2) Specialised. Attention here is devoted to the study of social skills in professional encounters. Such professionals will have particular vocational objectives which necessitate specialised forms of interaction. This type of specialised SST is now widely employed in nurse training, since it is recognised that nurses must possess certain interactive abilities in order to perform their duties effectively

(3) Remedial. In this context SST programmes are provided for those whose repertoire of effective social behaviours is inadequate for everyday life. The emphasis here is upon providing the individual with a knowledge of, and expertise in, relevant social skills.

It is with the latter context that this book is concerned. While

1

interest in the field of remedial SST has grown over the past few years, to date no book has examined the role of the psychiatric nurse in such training. Yet increasingly it is becoming clear that the psychiatric nurse has an important contribution to make to programmes of SST. In order to exploit fully their potential as social skills trainers, however, psychiatric nurses must have a full understanding of SST in terms of research, theory and practice. This is especially true since, as Phillips (1985) has pointed out:

> There is probably no aspect of the general delivery of mental health services — from intake through individual and group psychotherapy, in both in- and outpatient setting — that would fail to profit from a social skills approach.

The Nature of Social Skills

At this stage it is useful to examine exactly what is meant by the term 'social skill'. In one sense it would seem that this term is quite clear and needs no definition, since the reader will have understood what has been meant when social skill has been referred to in the above section. In this sense social skills are the skills employed when interacting with other people at an interpersonal level. However, this definition of social skills is not very illuminating since it refers to what social skills are *used for*, rather than what they *are*. Attempting to achieve conceptual clarification about the exact nature of social skills has in fact occupied the minds of many theorists in the past few years. The development of a social skills 'movement' has gradually evolved as a result of the search both for such conceptual clarification, and for a firm theoretical underpinning for SST.

As Hargie (1986) has illustrated, this systematic analysis and evaluation of social skills emanated from the study of motor skill performance. This latter field of study has been prevalent within psychology for well over a century, and as a result significant advances have been made into both identifying the central aspects of motor skill performance and training individuals to employ such skills effectively. Such knowledge has, amongst other outcomes, enabled machines to be designed in such a way as to facilitate the human operator and has resulted in the development of systematic and effective training methods for improving the performance of individuals on a wide range of motor tasks.

Given this in-depth knowledge of motor skill performance it was almost inevitable that eventually analogies would be drawn between the performance of motor skills and social skills. Welford (1980) identifies Crossman (1960) as first making the link between motor and social skill. Crossman collaborated with Michael Argyle, a social psychologist at Oxford University, and they carried out the first study of social skill designed specifically to investigate the similarities between man-machine and man-man interactions. Argyle (1972), in subsequent studies, developed these links into a model of motor skills which he argued could be applied directly to social skills. (This model will be described and evaluated in depth in Chapter 4.)

In investigating the nature of motor skill performance, Welford (1958) identified three main characteristics:

(1) They consist of an organised, co-ordinated activity in relation to an object or a situation, and therefore involve a whole chain of sensory, central and motor mechanisms which underlie performance
(2) They are learnt, in that the understanding of the event or performance is built up gradually with repeated experience
(3) They are serial in nature, involving the ordering and co-ordination of many different processes or actions in sequence.

Thus, skill basically involves the performance of goal-directed, co-ordinated behaviours that are learnt and improved upon with practice, with the outcome of the behaviours being constantly monitored to ascertain whether or not they are successful. In this way a skilled tennis player will have a goal (to win a point), will carry out co-ordinated behaviours (play shots), will evaluate these behaviours in relation to the goal (should he play more shots to his opponent's backhand?) and will improve his overall game with practice and experience. Similar patterns emerge in the performance of social skills. For example a young man may have a goal of getting a date with a female. To do so he will carry out certain behaviours (chatting up), will monitor the effectiveness of these behaviours and will usually improve his dating skills with experience.

Given these parallels between motor and social skills, various definitions of the term 'social skills' have been put forward by different theorists. Van Hasselt et al (1979) in evaluating such definitions identified three central aspects of social skill:

(1) Social skills are situation specific. Few, if any, interpersonal behaviours will have the same significance across situations and cultures. The meaning of any particular behaviour will vary according to the situation in which it occurs. Thus, prolonged eye contact may indicate great affection between two young lovers, or a prelude to physical violence between two young males

(2) Interpersonal effectiveness is judged on the basis of verbal and nonverbal response elements displayed by an individual. These responses are learned, and failure to learn social skills can result in social inadequacy

(3) The role of the other person is important, and interpersonal effectiveness should include the ability to behave without causing harm (verbal or physical) to others.

These three elements comprise the central core of social skill. A socially skilled individual will possess the ability to behave in an appropriate manner in any given situation. He or she can only be judged as socially skilled, however, on the basis of actual social performance. It is possible for someone to be familiar with the behaviours necessary to cope successfully in a given situation, in terms of being able to describe these behaviours, and yet still fail to put this knowledge into practice (through, for example, a high level of anxiety). Such a person would not be described as socially skilled. Thus, social skills refer to behaviour displayed by an individual.

In the light of this analysis, Hargie (1986) proposed a definition of social skill as 'a set of goal-directed, inter-related, situationally appropriate, social behaviours which can be learned and which are under the control of the individual'. This is the definition that we will employ in this book, since it has direct relevance to SST in the psychiatric setting. This can be illustrated by examining in more depth the six main features of the definition:

(1) Socially skilled behaviours are *goal-directed* and intentional. They are those behaviours that the individual employs in order to achieve a desired outcome, and are therefore purposeful behaviours, as opposed to chance or unintentional behaviours.

These goals may be subconscious during social interaction, and indeed this is a feature of skilled action. The skilled swimmer is not consciously aware of his goals as he swims through the water, but these goals will nevertheless determine his swimming behaviour. If he wants to swim faster he does not consciously think 'I want to swim faster, I must speed up my arm and leg movements'. Likewise, the socially skilled individual is not always consciously aware of his goals and does not consciously think 'I want to show him I am interested so I should nod my head, look at him, smile and look attentive'. Someone lacking social skill, however, may need to go through the process of consciously thinking about goals and related behaviours in order to become more skilled, just as the novice swimmer needs to learn how to achieve certain goals by performing certain swimming movements

(2) Social skill is defined in terms of overt *social behaviours* which are clearly observable to others. If someone always acts in a socially incompetent fashion, then he will be adjudged to be socially inadequate, regardless of how good he may be at theorising about how to behave. Thus, actual behaviour is the main defining feature of skilled performance. Skilled behaviour is hierarchically organised with larger sequences (such as being interviewed) being comprised of smaller units (such as sitting appropriately, engaging in eye contact, answering questions etc.). In order to successfully assimilate the large sequences it is therefore necessary to learn first to utilise each of the smaller units. Again, this is similar to motor skill performance. For example, in order to learn how to drive a car it is first necessary to learn how to switch on the engine, change the gears, use the brake and so on.

(3) The behaviours employed must be *situationally appropriate*. The same set of behaviours may be regarded as social skill in one situation yet be indicative of lack of skill in another. For example, singing *risque* songs, telling 'blue' jokes and using crude language may be appropriate at an all-male drinking session after a rugby match. The same behaviour would, however, be frowned upon if displayed in mixed company during a meal at a high class restaurant! It is therefore essential to be able to evaluate which behaviours to employ in various situations. This is an aspect of skill which is lacking amongst social inadequates, who may either have a fixed set of responses and

be unable to vary these, or may tend to 'say the right thing at the wrong time'. As before, there are close parallels here with motor skills. The skilled footballer needs to be able to take into account prevailing conditions (wind, rain etc.) when deciding which moves to make. Furthermore, quite often skilled club players find it difficult to adapt to the new demands made when they move up to play at international level — in other words they may not have the necessary skill to adjust to the new situation

(4) Social skills consist of a number of *inter-related* social behaviours, that is behaviours that are combined to achieve a common goal. Someone wishing to provide reward to another will smile, use head nods, look at the other person and make an appropriate statement such as 'That's very interesting'. (The skill of rewarding is reviewed in Chapter 9.) In this instance, all of these behaviours are inter-related in that they are all indicative of the skill of rewarding. However, if someone does not look at us, yawns, uses no head nods yet says 'That's very interesting', these behaviours would be contradictory rather than complementary and the person would not be using the skill of rewarding very successfully. In the use of motor skills, behaviours are also inter-related so that the car driver needs to synchronise his use of the clutch, accelerator, gear lever and steering wheel simultaneously

(5) Social skills are comprised of *learned* behaviours. All social behaviour is learned: we know that if children are reared in isolation they do not develop socially acceptable behaviour patterns. Indeed, there is evidence to suggest that the degree of deprivation of appropriate learning experiences from other humans will differentially affect the social behaviours of individuals. Children from socially deprived home backgrounds tend to develop unacceptable social behaviours, whereas children from culturally richer home environments tend to develop more appropriate social behaviour patterns (Rutter, 1972).

These findings are in line with the social learning theory put forward by Bandura (1971). This theory purports that all behaviour, with the exception of elementary reflexes (such as eye blinking or coughing), is learned. Such learning, he argues, involves the observation of other people, and modelling and imitating the behaviour of significant others, such as parents, peers, siblings, teachers, film stars etc. Thus, the individual watches how others behave and then imitates this behaviour. Such a process occurs from an early age, so that children often walk, talk and behave like their same-sex parent. At a later stage, however, children usually begin to use as models other people who are more significant in their lives. As the individual tries out various types of behaviour they will receive reinforcement from others, and will tend to employ more frequently those behaviours that are rewarded, while employing less frequently those that are punished. In this way the social repertoire of the individual is developed

(6) The final element of social skill, which is also an important facet of Bandura's social learning theory, is the degree of cognitive *control* that the individual has over his behaviour. Thus, for example, a socially inadequate person may have learned how to use certain behaviours, but may not have developed the necessary thought processes to control the utilisation of these behaviours. The timing of social responses is crucial, in that knowing *when* to say or do something is as important as knowing *how* to say or do it. The cognitive capacity of the individual will also influence his ability to learn new skills, thus where someone is suffering from a severe cognitive impairment it is unlikely that SST will be effective or indeed appropriate. The greater an individual's cognitive capacity, the faster he will be able to process information. Thus, a Formula One racing driver will have a much greater capacity for processing information about road conditions etc. and so will be able to respond more quickly during races than would an average motorist. Similarly a highly socially skilled individual will be able to process social information rapidly and make appropriate responses. In both instances, the degree of cognitive control has a direct bearing upon skilled performance. This is particularly important since skilled performance requires the operation of a sequence of behaviours in rapid succession. Thus, a car driver has to carry out a set of behaviours in a particular sequence in order to start the engine and move the car (turn the key in the ignition, press the clutch, engage the gear etc). Likewise, many social actions require behaviours to be performed in sequence. Morris (1971), for example, has identified the following sequence for courtship: eye to body; eye to eye; voice to voice; hand to hand; arm to

shoulder; arm to waist; mouth to mouth; hand to head; hand to body; mouth to breast; hand to genitals; genitals to genitals. Being able to carry out such sequences effectively requires a degree of cognitive potential which, if absent, makes social learning impossible.

As this analysis of social skill indicates, there are many similarities between social skills and motor skills, and it is therefore useful to conceptualise interpersonal communication as a type of skilled performance (there are also some important differences between these two sets of skills and these will be discussed in Chapter 4). The most promising aspect of this approach is that it emphasises the fact that social skills involve the learning of certain behaviours. This means that it is possible to teach such skills to certain individuals who demonstrate deficits in social performance. Hence the recent interest in SST as a method for remediating the social deficits of some psychiatric patients.

SST and Psychiatric Nursing

This book is designed to provide the nurse with an overview of the social skills approach. In Chapter 2 we discuss the types of patient likely to benefit from SST. This is related to an analysis of how interpersonal failures can be the consequence of other disorders (such as anxiety) or how, in turn, social skills deficits may lead to, or be considered a precipitatory factor of, certain psychiatric conditions. This chapter also examines the nature of these social skill deficits in terms of a continuum of complexity ranging from problems in basic life skills (as displayed by many institutionalised long-stay patients) to problems in larger social skill elements (as often encountered by patients in acute/short-stay wards and day hospitals).

Chapter 3 examines the role of the psychiatric nurse in relation to the way in which psychiatric disorders have been treated in the past and how this treatment/management has changed in recent years. In particular, the developing and evolving role of the psychiatric nurse is discussed with reference to the demands brought about by recent innovations such as SST. This focuses upon changes in the nurse training syllabus and growing recognition of the need to move from a traditional generic role to a more specialised role. In Chapter 4 the theoretical framework for SST is provided in terms of a model of interpersonal communication, which develops and extends a similar model used in the analysis of motor skill performance.

In Chapter 5 the procedures involved in setting up an SST programme in a psychiatric context are presented. This will incorporate sections on identification and assessment of deficits, goal setting, sensitisation, modelling, practice and feedback. These aspects are complemented in Chapter 6, where some of the issues involved in actually implementing SST are discussed, such as liaison with other professionals, group versus individual approaches to training, differences in approach and objectives with long-stay as opposed to short-stay/acute patients, ethical considerations and evaluation of the effectiveness of SST.

Chapters 7, 8 and 9 are devoted to an analysis of the main social skills that have been identified to date, namely nonverbal communication, greetings and partings, and self-disclosure (Chapter 7); questioning, explaining, assertiveness and interacting in groups (Chapter 8); listening, reflecting, showing empathy and reinforcing (Chapter 9). Exercises relating to each of these skills are presented in Chapter 10. Together, then, these four chapters provide the nurse with useful resource material for running an SST programme. Finally, Chapter 11 teases out the central issues raised throughout the book and ties these together.

Overall, therefore, the book should be of value to nurses who are interested in becoming involved in SST as a method of remediation. Throughout the book we have attempted to confine our use of references to central texts, and we would recommend that some of the references used in each chapter be consulted by the nurse wishing to obtain a more in-depth knowledge of the many facets of this training approach.

2 THE PSYCHIATRIC PATIENT AND SOCIAL SKILLS TRAINING

Although social skills deficits may be experienced by a variety of people, empirical studies have shown that many psychiatric patients are, for numerous reasons, socially inadequate in certain situations (Libet and Lewinsohn, 1973). Generally speaking, it is not the type of social skills deficit that distinguishes psychiatric patients from the non-psychiatric population, but the degree to which the social inadequacy disrupts the person's social life. However, the distinction in social skills deficits between the psychiatric and non-psychiatric population is often considered to be both subjective and nebulous.

This chapter will identify psychiatric patients who might benefit from SST. Firstly, however, the acquisition of social skills will be examined, followed by a review of factors that may either impede acquisition or prevent one from using them effectively. The chapter will end with a brief review of literature concerning the effectiveness of SST in psychiatry.

Social Skills Acquisition

In discussing problems in social skill acquisition it is firstly necessary to outline briefly the theories behind the acquisition of social skills. Although there is comparatively little direct evidence available, it is generally acknowledged that social skills are acquired gradually throughout childhood and adolescence, continuing into adulthood. As discussed in Chapter 1, according to Bandura (1971) such social learning involves the modelling on and imitation of others. In his studies he described the influence of observational or vicarious learning (termed 'modelling') on social behaviour and demonstrated its effect in a large number of studies. Children, adolescents and even adults, he purports, develop new competencies to cope with social situations by observing how live models around them perform socially. In addition to the use of live models, learning can also be accomplished by using portrayed models such as on television and films, and symbolic models such as idealised, elaborate verbal descriptions of the conduct of another person (e.g. a good Christian or an ideal employee). Thus social skill knowledge may be acquired initially without personal learning experience in the relevant situations. The repetition of social behaviour, Bandura argues, requires reinforcement, where appropriate behaviour is encouraged and rewarded and inappropriate behaviour is discouraged. This process begins very early in life. Even during early infancy it is apparent that rudimentary social behaviours can be developed and maintained by their reinforcing consequences. If social behaviour in a given situation is reinforced through some positive outcome, it will not only tend to recur, but will also change and become more effective over time. If a social behaviour, however, is repeatedly attempted but does not lead to some positive consequence, especially during the earlier stages of learning, it is likely to be extinguished and cease to be exhibited. Hence the use or denial of reinforcement may play a dominant role in the development of an individual's social skill repertoire.

In addition to modelling and reinforcement, Trower et al (1978) advocate the importance of other factors in the acquisition of appropriate social skills. Firstly, the opportunity to observe and practise appropriate behaviour in a range of situations. While verbally presented instructions or examples may provide initial insight into socially skilled behaviour, observing a model actually exhibiting the skill component and affording the client the opportunity to practise, enables greater understanding of the social behaviour. Allowing the client to practise in a range of situations permits generalisations to be made, whereby newly acquired social skills can be employed successfully under conditions different from those surrounding the initial learning of the skill. It is not possible for clients in SST to rehearse every social eventuality, instead they must be able to generalise their use of newly acquired skills, tailoring them to meet the demands of specific social situations. If, for example, SST phsyically takes place in a hospital, but the real problem situations occur in a client's home or workplace, the client must exhibit his or her new ways of dealing with the natural environment situation in which it actually occurs.

Secondly, Trower et al (1978) highlight the importance of the development of cognitive abilities in the acquisition of effective social skills. These include the way in which the person thinks about himself and his problems, his cognitive appraisal of the situation and his ability to generate alternative solutions and evaluate possible outcomes of various strategies. Although the processes are not clear, it is generally accepted that cognitive abilities occur through the combined influence of innate potential and environmental experience. Deprivation studies show that an unstimulating environment, and in particular undifferentiated stimulation which lacks meaning with regard to the child's own responses, can adversely affect the development of cognitive abilities. The cognitive abilities of children have received much interest in recent years. Whilst developmental psychologists such as Piaget claim that cognitive abilities develop in a series of stages in children and that certain abilities are impossible if the child has not reached the appropriate age, studies by Bryant (1974) show that abilities such as empathy and making logical inferences occur much earlier than Piaget claims. Therefore the stage in life at which cognitive abilities develop and the extent to which they develop both play an important part in the acquisition of appropriate social skills.

Finally, Trower et al postulate that the innate potential of the individual (nature as opposed to nurture) may be significant in the acquisition of appropriate social skills. The part genetic influences play is uncertain and at times difficult to differentiate from other factors. Studies suggest that no one influence is primarily responsible but rather the factors influencing social skills acquisition are inter-related.

Problems in Social Skill Acquisition

On the basis of theory it would seem reasonable to accept that problems in social skills acquisition can result from either a disruption in the learning of an appropriate range of social skills, or from factors preventing the person from using the social skills that have been learned. In addition, Argyle (1972) suggests that the failure of social behaviour may be due to the person deliberately producing certain social signals in a bid for help or sympathy. Disruption in the learning of appropriate social skills may occur for a variety of reasons:

(1) Absence of suitable social skills models (e.g. parents) may lead to the individual being unable to observe appropriate social skills

(2) Inappropriate or poor social skills models can result in the acquisition of less desirable social skills. This area has been explored in the development of psychiatric illnesses such as psychopathy and inadequate personality

(3) Lack of reinforcement may lead to appropriate social skills being discouraged

(4) Appropriate social skills may be acquired, but only in a limited range of situations

(5) Arrest in development of cognitive abilities can result in the individual being unable to process information and make inferences. This may be due to certain environmental deprivations, as suggested by Rutter (1972), who stated that poverty of stimulation can have negative consequences for cognitive development. Cognitive abilities may also be arrested by disruptions in mental development caused by physical conditions such as brain trauma, rubella during pregnancy and hereditary conditions such as Down's syndrome. These latter conditions are prevalent within the field of the mentally handicapped.

Irrespective of the reasons why appropriate social skills are not learned, deficits can not only lead to a variety of social difficulties for the individual (i.e. inability to make friends easily or to cope with interviews), but may also result in social isolation, withdrawal, loneliness and social anxiety. This may, in extreme cases, ultimately lead to the person being unable to cope socially, resulting in the development of psychiatric problems. Unfortunately, a vicious cycle may evolve whereby the psychiatric condition emerges as a consequence of inadequate social skills; the psychiatric condition may in turn enhance the patient's social skill inadequacy; and so a continuous cycle of events is created (see Figure 2.1).

Failure to perform social skills, on the other hand, may be due to the fact that an appropriate range of social skills has been attained, but for some reason the individual is temporarily (in some instances permanently) unable to make full use of them. This may characteristically be witnessed in certain psychiatric conditions where the psychological and sometimes physical manifestations of the condition inhibit the person from making satisfactory social relationships, or from dealing with particular social situations. Abnormalities in areas such as thought, speech, perception, mood and behaviour may severely restrict the patient's social skills reper-

Figure 2.1: Social Skills Deficits as a (a) Consequence and (b) as a
Precipitator of Psychiatric Disorder

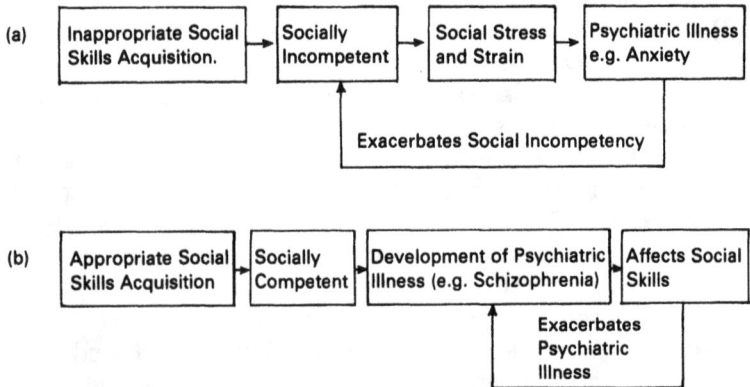

(a)

| Inappropriate Social Skills Acquisition. | → | Socially Incompetent | → | Social Stress and Strain | → | Psychiatric Illness e.g. Anxiety |

Exacerbates Social Incompetency

(b)

| Appropriate Social Skills Acquisition | → | Socially Competent | → | Development of Psychiatric Illness (e.g. Schizophrenia) | → | Affects Social Skills |

Exacerbates
Psychiatric
Illness

toire. This, unfortunately, often hinders the development of a
therapeutic nurse-patient relationship, and clearly illustrates the
necessity for nurses to be both socially skilled themselves and
knowledgeable in the field of SST. It is salient at this point to note
that many conditions found within the general sphere of nursing
have concomitant psychological consequences that may result in
the patient experiencing certain social skill deficits. Examples
include the stroke patient with aphasia and partial paralysis, and
the patient with a permanent colostomy. In both conditions the
patient may experience difficulty with self-image and self-
confidence, particularly when interacting with others. Thus,
although this book is most relevant to the psychiatrically ill patient,
the principles of SST can also be applied to other areas of nursing
where social skills deficits exist.

In addition to psychiatric illnesses impeding social skills performance, the environment in which one finds oneself can also
affect behaviour. The effects of institutionalisation on the
behaviour of the individual has been widely studied and work by
Wing and Brown (1970) and Barton (1976) vividly describe how
individuals with a previously appropriate social skill reportoire are
severely affected by the institution in which they live. Not only are
the individuals psychologically affected by being socially withdrawn, lacking in spontaneity and submissive, but they also change
physically in their posture, facial expression and dress. Institutions,

therefore, because of their unique social culture and the restrictive learning environment inhibit patients from using their full range of social skills.

The effects of institutionalisation on the patient's psychiatric illness serve to exacerbate further the primary condition (see Figure 2.2). In some instances the effects may be so severe that they may even supersede the patient's primary illness. This is of great significance to the psychiatric nurse when planning patient care. It would be counterproductive, in an SST programme, if the patient was placed in an environment that not only restricted the practice of appropriate social skills but also actively discouraged it. This may be due to lack of reinforcement, or the result of poor modelling of social skills by both patients and staff. For example Coulthard (1984) in studying ordinary conversation, identified that 'caring staff' may be more socially incompetent than the patient. In describing ordinary conversation, Coulthard referred to 'the way control of topic passes from one participant to another and the way in which speakers produce coherent discourse with each successive utterance topically relevant to the one that preceded it'. Coulthard, by observing a conversational interview between a consultant psychiatrist and a person suffering from schizophrenia, concluded that in many ways it was the psychiatrist who was socially deviant, failing to respond appropriately to any-

Figure 2.2: Effects of Psychiatric Illness and the Environment on Social Skills

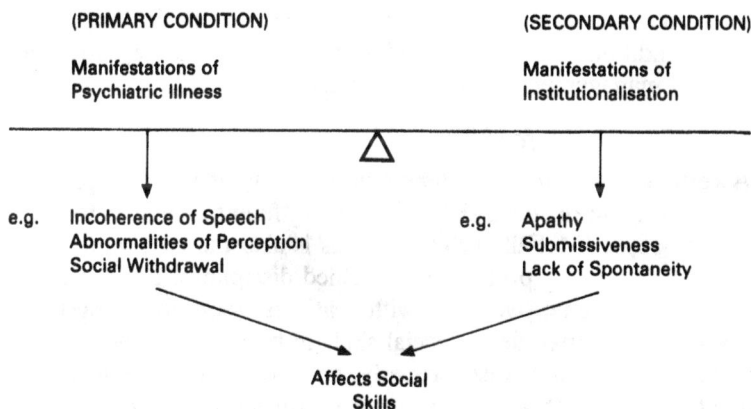

(PRIMARY CONDITION)	(SECONDARY CONDITION)
Manifestations of Psychiatric Illness	Manifestations of Institutionalisation

e.g. Incoherence of Speech   Abnormalities of Perception   Social Withdrawal

e.g. Apathy   Submissiveness   Lack of Spontaneity

Affects Social Skills

thing the patient said! For many patients interaction can be a problem, particularly in continued care wards. Conversing with staff who also display inappropriate social skills does little to enhance the patient's interactional competency.

In conclusion, deficits in the social skills repertoire of people who suffer from psychiatric illness arise for several reasons. They are not only a consequence of a psychiatric condition, but can also occur independently and even precipitate psychological disorders.

Psychiatric Patients who would Benefit from SST

Having examined the cause and effect phenomenon of social skills deficits and psychological disorders, the psychiatric conditions which would benefit from SST will now be analysed more closely.

It must be emphasised that although classifications of different psychiatric illnesses are included within this text, it is done to help the reader clarify the situation in which SST may be used. The authors advocate moving from diagnostic criteria as a means of determining the suitability of SST to assessing the individual needs of the patient irrespective of medical diagnosis. As stated by Marzillier and Winter (1978) 'the inclusion of any individual in a programme of social skills training does not follow from any particular description or psychiatric diagnosis in the traditional sense. Rather, it is determined by a careful behavioural analysis which indicates that poor social skills may be giving rise to psychological discomfort.' Such meticulous assessment of the patient and selection of a suitable means of treatment will help to ensure that SST is not used indiscriminately as a panacea for particular psychiatric conditions, but rather is identified as the most appropriate form of management for a specific individual.

Social Skills and Life Skills

Ascertaining the appropriateness of SST may at times be problematic as the term social skills can have different meanings for different people (McFall, 1982) and this is also the case within the psychiatric nursing profession and allied disciplines. For example, nursing personnel working with patients requiring long-term hospitalisation may define social skills in basic terms, such as the ability to dress and wash properly, and others may see it as the ability to cope with a range of social activities essential to everyday life, such as travelling by bus, shopping and so on. Conversely many consider these to be 'coping' or 'daily living' skills as distinct from social skills.

If, however, one adopts the premise proposed by Argyle (1972) that social skills can be hierarchically organised, with large social elements being comprised of smaller behavioural units, cognisance must be taken of the basic coping or daily living skills and the role they play in developing social competence. While the hierarchical principle, because of its simplicity, may assist greater understanding of the social skills concept, it can also be misleading by depicting some social skill units to be more complex than others. For this reason we have adopted a columnar representation to portray not only the different elements and units of social skills, but also the relationship between personal and interpersonal skills (see Figure 2.3).

An understanding of the relationship between the different skills is essential if SST programmes are to be effective. It is rather futile, for example, to devise an SST programme to help promote an individual's eye contact, when their fundamental skills like personal cleanliness are inadequate. An SST programme, like any nursing care plan, must meet the patient's needs in terms of priority, ensuring that the personal skills at the base of the column are adequate before progression is made. In order for a person to master the more complex socially skilled responses he must first command the smaller behavioural units. The distinction between social skills and daily living skills is a tenuous and arbitrary one. Although many exponents do make the distinction, there is a growing awareness by some, such as Westland (1980) and Van Den Pol et al (1981) that a social behavioural approach can be used to improve a patient's basic coping or daily living skills. Since daily living skills play an integral part in creating a sound foundation upon which effective social skills can be acquired, cognisance will be taken of both when identifying the type of psychiatric patient who would benefit from SST.

Types of Psychiatric Patient

Patients experiencing deficits at the bottom of the column (as depicted in Figure 2.3) are characteristically seen in the long-stay wards of psychiatric hospitals and in certain sections of the mentally handicapped population. Skills deficits in these areas can be the result of a chronic mental disorder (e.g. chronic schizophrenia)

Figure 2.3: Columnar Representation of Social and Life Skills

Making Friends	
Apologising	Larger
Dating	Social Skill
Being Interviewed	Elements

Self Disclosure — Opening		
Explaining — Closing		Smaller
Questioning — Listening		Social Skills
Nonverbal Communication — Reflecting		Units
Reinforcing — Asserting		

Eating Etiquette	
Dress Sense	Daily
Ability to Dress Self	Living
Toilet Etiquette	Skills
Ability to Wash Self	

but often are the product of institutionalisation. The deficits observed in these types of patient are frequently the most extreme forms of social inadequacy and may affect the individual physically, psychologically and socially. Social inadequacies include irrational, meaningless and sometimes antisocial behaviour, inability to attend to personal hygiene and dress, lack of empathy and spontaneity and so on. Many of the deficits resulting from institutionalisation, like social skills, are themselves learned.

Lack of appropriate social skills, as portrayed in the higher sections of the column, has been implicated in a wide range of psychiatric conditions. Patients suffering from schizophrenia exhibit many social peculiarities including: odd untidy appearance; inability to wear clothes well; adopting unsuitable proximities (either too close or too far); inappropriate orientation, poor eye contact; constantly averting gaze; flattening of emotion; incongruous gestures, postures and expressions; perceptual insensitivity; and often rambling, incoherent and poorly synchronised speech. They experience great difficulty in initiating conversation and when engaged in interaction often fail to reciprocate, with resultant breakdown in rapport. A failure of persistent goal-directed behaviour is often evident, for instance the behaviour of a person suffering from schizophrenia often appears to be lacking in purpose and intention.

Social isolation, therefore, may not only occur as a direct result of the schizophrenic condition, but can also be exacerbated by the caring staff (including the psychiatric nurse) failing to communicate with the patient because of the seemingly unrewarding nature of the interaction. The very nature of a schizophrenic illness, however, (i.e. affecting the patient's cognitive abilities) may warrant the use of treatments other than SST. Notice must be taken of the patient's participation in treatment and, bearing in mind that a treatment contract is entered into by both the patient and the nurse (see Chapters 5 and 6 for sections on contract formation), any condition that prevents him understanding the SST concept may necessitate other approaches.

In reactive depression social skill inadequacies, including poor voice quality, lack of spontaneity in conversation, dulling of emotional reponses and loss of interest in friends and social life, are often apparent. Depressives have a lower opinion of themselves than is warranted and are completely lacking in self-confidence. Studies by Libet and Lewinsohn (1973) on the inter-relationship between depression and social difficulties and by Wells et al (1979) postulated that patients with reactive depression are frequently fraught by inter-personal difficulties. Consequently, they suggest, treatment techniques aimed at directly teaching appropriate social skills behaviour may be an important approach in the treatment of depression.

Socially anxious patients, on the other hand, may not lack in spontaneity or appear socially withdrawn, but conversely may be over-talkative, continually disclosing their emotions and physical state. They can be seen to be in a state of tension in social situations from their strained faces, trembling hands, tense posture, rapid breathing and poorly controlled gestures. In addition they are often tense, irritable and easily upset. The inability to interact effectively may serve to enhance the anxiety and so further exacerbate their primary condition. Since they frequently disclose negative information about themselves, interaction can be unrewarding for the nurse and may even lead to the patient being avoided.

There also exist within the psychiatrically ill population forms of social inadequacy that are not easily classified into diagnostic categories and are thus considered to be separate conditions. These conditions are often ill-defined and little consensus exists as to what exactly constitutes a condition of social inadequacy. Despite this vagueness, certain social skills deficits, as identified by Trower et al (1978), predominate, including lack of assertiveness, little variation of facial expression, poor eye contact, closed posture, slow monotonous voice and lack of continuity and spontaneity of conversation. Psychopathic individuals might also be included in this section; while lacking the usual symptoms of neurosis or psychosis, they are disturbed primarily in the social sphere. The main characteristics include impulsiveness, unrestrained aggression or sexuality, lack of conscience, and lack of sympathy, affection or consideration for others. Although the aetiology is unsure, it is firmly believed that such undesirable social skills may be the result of inappropriate or poor social models early in the individual's life. The area of social inadequacy (and to a lesser degree psychopathy) and SST has received particular attention in recent years. In accepting the view that social inadequacy can be treated directly by training the patient in the social skills in which he is deficient, precipitatory factors causing the psychiatric conditions can be minimised or removed.

Although most literature concentrates on the application of SST to the conditions mentioned above, there is a growing awareness that the principles of SST may be applied to other psychiatric conditions where social difficulties are encountered by patients. For example, studies by O'Leary et al (1976) which examined social skills acquisition in alcoholics, concluded that pre-alcoholic male teenagers are less socially skilled than light or non-drinkers of the same age, and that alcoholics show a lack of appropriate interpersonal coping behaviours. Thus O'Leary et al recommended that 'therapeutic interventions aimed at the development or expansion of the alcoholic's social skills repertoire would provide the alcoholic with socially adaptive alternative responses to drinking in settings previously related to alcohol consumption'. Pillay and Crisp (1977) identified social isolation and low self-esteem in anorectics, and Stonehill and Crisp (1977) noticed that following traditional forms of treatment anorexic patients often became socially anxious. SST directed at ameliorating the social difficulties of patients suffering from anorexia nervosa would hopefully lead to a greater degree of recovery.

The Effectiveness of SST

Whilst this chapter has sought to identify the types of psychiatrically ill individuals who might benefit from SST, it must be remembered that the concept is still relatively new to the psychiatric field. Consequently the appropriateness, effectiveness and mode of application of the social approach in the management of many psychological problems has yet to be fully determined and warrants further investigation and research. The effectiveness of SST has been demonstrated with such diverse groups as children who evidence poor interpersonal skills (Panepinto, 1976), couples with marital difficulties (Fensterheim, 1972), individuals who frequently engage in aggressive behaviours (Foy et al, 1975), and sexual offenders (Marshall and McKnight, 1975) as well as arsonists (Rice and Chaplin, 1979) who demonstrate poor interpersonal skills.

Studies conducted into the effectiveness of SST with psychiatric patients have tended to demonstrate that this training method is effective in that patients display improved social competence immediately following training. However, results are more equivocal with regard to the long-term retention of social skills in follow-up studies of SST. Argyle et al (1974) carried out detailed studies on the components of social interaction. They used SST techniques to improve the social repertoire of socially inadequate patients. As well as practising specific difficult situations (such as job intervews), the subjects were taught to improve their posture, eye contact, gestures, expression and voice control. Results suggested that SST produced significant improvement in social interaction, with some improvement in psychiatric symptoms.

Modelling with practice and reinforcement to train neurotic patients was used by Ullrich de Muynck and Ullrich (1972).

Subjects were taught to respond more confidently in a variety of difficult social situations. The experimental group showed significantly less insecurity (fear of failure, inability to refuse) than the control group after 30 hours of treatment, and this was maintained at 6-month follow-up. Sarason and Ganzer (1973) used modelling, practice and discussion to teach juvenile delinquent boys appropriate new responses to difficult social situations where their previous responses had been inappropriate and had led to trouble. Themes such as asking personal advice, resisting group pressure, handling authority, and coping with job interviews and work situations were practised. Significant improvement in the social interaction of the boys was noted. Studies by Gutride et al (1973) on acute chronic psychiatric in-patients were carried out to assess a form of SST which they labelled Structured Learning Therapy. In their studies Gutride et al sought to effect a change in the social behaviour of predominantly schizophrenic patients. The studies showed Structured Learning Therapy to produce a significant improvement in both acute and chronic patients, compared with a no-treatment control group and an inactive treatment control group.

Marzillier et al (1976) carried out a study on socially inadequate psychiatric patients where the results showed that SST led to a significant improvement in the patient's social life, which was maintained at 6-month follow-up. In their study of the long-term effects of group and individual SST with alcoholics, Oei and Jackson (1980) compared SST to traditional forms of treatment. Social skills trained subjects improved significantly more than subjects receiving traditional forms of treatment on all measures throughout the 12-week periods. Furthermore, subjects receiving group SST scored consistently better than those receiving individual SST.

Shepherd and Spence (1983) in their review conclude that 'SST is clearly effective in producing limited changes, in specific targets, evaluated over short periods of time. Whether it is also effective in producing rather wider, more 'clinical' changes which are generalised and stable, seems more doubtful'. They also point out that this problem of generalisation and retention following intervention is common across many therapeutic techniques, and recommend that trainers in SST pay more attention to methods whereby skills learned during SST can be transferred across time and situations (see Chapter 5). Where specific attention is given during SST to these issues of generalisation and retention of social skills, results have proved to be very favourable. Thus, Monti et al (1982) report retention of social skills at both 6- and 10-month follow-up intervals, and attribute this to their 'special emphasis on promoting the generalization of social competence'. In particular, they emphasise the importance of homework assignments in making the content of SST *directly* relevant to the social difficulties faced by patients, and of ensuring that the SST programme is of a significant duration to ensure worthwhile results. This latter point is important, since programmes of SST tend to vary markedly in both length and content, and this makes comparisons between research studies very difficult. Suffice it to say that while existing findings suggest that generalisation of social skills is not always achieved following SST, there is evidence to indicate that it is possible to obtain such generalisation (Field and Test, 1975; Goldsmith and McFall, 1975).

This selective review of research studies provides encouraging evidence that SST can provide improvements in the social behaviour of psychiatric patients. Research into the use of SST with psychiatric patients can be summarised in the words of Van Hasselt et al (1978) who in a review of research concluded that patients 'can be trained to perform more competently in inter-personal skill situations that have been distressing for them in the past. However, more clinical research is needed to verify this contention and to maximise the potential gains from skill acquisition strategies'. Little has changed to alter this conclusion.

Overview

In this chapter the development of and problems in social skills acquisition and the types of psychiatric patient who might benefit from SST have been described. It is worth emphasising here that although many psychiatric patients may experience social skills deficits, SST is but one approach in helping them with their problems. If properly assessed, patients can present other features that negate the use of the SST approach. SST, therefore, must be selected carefully and tailored to suit the individual needs of the patient. Given a careful selection of patients, and a well structured patient programme, it does seem that SST can be beneficial in improving the social competence of patients in the short- and the long-term.

3 THE PSYCHIATRIC NURSE AND SOCIAL SKILLS TRAINING

The role of the psychiatric nurse, like the management of mental disorders, has evolved markedly over the past few centuries, but particularly within the past three decades. The psychiatric nurse in both hospital and community has become increasingly involved in areas that have, in the past, been the responsibility of the medical profession. This trend is the result of a number of factors, including a change in the treatment philosophy of psychiatric conditions and the growth in the specialist expertise of the nurse.

In this chapter the role of the psychiatric nurse will be examined in relation to the way in which psychiatric disorders have been managed in the past and how these treatments have changed in recent years. In particular, the developing and evolving role of the psychiatric nurse will be discussed with reference to the demands brought about by recent innovations such as SST. This will entail an indepth description of the various factors that influence psychiatric nursing, including nurse education and the search for professional status.

Historical Review of Psychiatry

The role of the psychiatric nurse is determined by the changing patterns of psychiatry. In order to appreciate more fully the evolving role of the psychiatric nurse, it is firstly salutary to take a cursory look at the historical development of psychiatric care. Psychiatry, like the field of psychiatric nursing, is a relatively new area of study. While the areas of medical research, study and practice can be traced to biblical times, psychiatry and related disciplines only really date back to the last century. Facilities and care of the mentally ill prior to the drastic reforms of the nineteenth century were totally inadequate, often creating conditions in which the insane were treated with appalling neglect and revolting cruelty. During this period, people considered insane, crazy or lunatic were commonly managed at home by family members. Owing to their bizzare, antisocial behaviour and the absence of cure, they were often locked away from the time the problem became apparent until the time of their natural death. This 'natural death' was hastened by the fact that the imprisoned individual was deprived of many of the life-support systems available to other people in society, e.g. friends, employment and leisure. Those who could not be managed at home were admitted to hospital and treated alongside the physically ill in the local infirmaries. Many of the mentally insane, however, who were not accommodated by the family or hospital, were left to roam the countryside, retaining their liberty unless they became dangerous or likely to cause a public disturbance. Hence the emphasis was on protection of the state rather than the care of the insane. The 'roaming lunatics' joined the scores of wandering people and no distinction was made between lunatics, beggars or vagrants. Some of these wanderers were permitted to roam the streets and beg, but others were whipped and ejected from towns.

Societal attitudes towards the mentally ill during the medieval period was rather changeable. Those who showed symptoms of mental illness were often considered to be possessed of devils. Treatment that consisted of exorcism was replaced by persecution as the belief in, and fear of, witches increased. Many thousands of people who would now be considered mentally ill, died as a result of the purges against witches during this period. Gradually, however, attitudes changed and some religious orders began to care for the mentally ill. It was during this era that the first recognised institution designed solely to cater for the mentally insane was formed. St Mary's of Bethelem, though founded in 1272, was not given to the city of London by Henry VIII as a hospital for lunatics until 1547. This was the first hospital in Western Europe established exclusively for the mentally ill. Many patients were constantly bound in chains and fetters and they were provided with straw beds to sleep on. Recommendations were made that the patient should be closely guarded in a chamber where there was little light, and should be kept in permanent fear of his 'keeper'. Lunatic patients were considered a source of entertainment, with people paying to see these apparently fascinating spectacles. Although management was primarily custodial in nature, certain 'treatments' were practised, including semi-starvation, beatings, purgation and bleeding. Treatments were often punitive in nature with occasional fatal consequences. As a result of mechanical restraint and mal-treatment, violence and aggression within these establishments was not uncommon. In order to gain patient submission, more severe and grotesque methods of restraint were used. Such practices continued right through to the end of the eighteenth century.

Reforms in Mental Health Care

William Turke, disillusioned by the prevailing treatments, initiated changes in the care of the mentally ill in 1796. Turke, who founded the York Retreat, based his reforms on the work carried out by French physician Philippe Pinel in Bicêtre Hospital, Paris. Pinel, convinced that patients need not be chained or fettered, introduced light, fresh air, cleanliness, workshops and promenades. For the first time patients were housed in different wards depending on their degree of mental disturbance, with separate accommodation for those who were also physically sick. Like Pinel's venture, Turke's reforms in the York Retreat, emphasising a milder and more appropriate system, were considered to be highly successful. When freed from their chains, far from attacking their liberator, patients became much less violent and more amenable. The traditional medical treatments for mental disorder, for example bleeding, purgatives and so on, were now regarded as of little use.

Following Turke's reforms, Sir George Onesiphorus Paul of Gloucester lobbied the Secretary of State in 1806 proposing the establishment of Asylums for the Insane at public expense. An act was passed in 1808 with the purpose of providing 'better care and maintenance of lunatics being paupers or criminals in England'. The act empowered (but did not compel) the county magistrates to build asylums. Compulsion followed in an act of 1845. Large isolated hospitals were built as a result (the first opened in 1812), many of which are still in use. Although the 1808 parliamentary act provided institutions in which the mentally ill could be managed, it did little initially to enhance the quality of the overall care delivered to the patient. As a result of overcrowding, insufficient and untrained staff, the conditions in 'psychiatric institutions' in England came under scrutiny. Physical restraints, both mechanical and manual, were frequently used, excessive emetics and purgatives were employed and many deaths as a result of cruelty and neglect went unreported. Following investigations into maltreatments, courses of instruction in psychiatry were introduced for medical staff. This enabled doctors to have a greater insight into psychiatric disorders, resulting in more humane methods of management. Treatments throughout this period remained primarily medically orientated. This was due to the fact that administers were medical men, who sought physical causes for psychological disorders. The re-emergence of physical treatments was also due to growth in clinical knowledge and technical expertise.

Introduction of Therapeutic Forms of Treatment

There was at this time, however, increasing interest in a different school of thought. Sigmund Freud, together with Joseph Breuer, Pierre Janet and others, developed a psychotherapeutic approach, called psychoanalysis, for the treatment of mental disorder. The exponents of this approach believed that the behavioural disturbances and distress of the patient were due to the presence of powerful psychological forces, both conscious and unconscious, within the mind of the individual. Therefore, they advocated that treatment should be directed towards identifying these conflicts, demonstrating their presence, analysing their meaning and helping the patient to resolve them and replace them with more adaptive behaviour. Although Freud's theory may not greatly have affected the medical philosophy of treatment at that time, it has in one form or another, influenced much of modern thinking in psychiatry.

Although mechanical restraint was employed less frequently from the late nineteenth century onwards, restraint of patients did persist through administration of chemicals. Bromides were introduced in 1857 and barbituates in 1903. Both, although effective in controlling disturbed behaviour, were purely symptomatic in their action, having no direct effect on the cause of illness. They were nevertheless considered a major breakthrough in the treatment of the mentally ill, and heralded the beginning of an era that saw the introduction of more therapeutic forms of treatment. Instead of merely providing a custodial regime, more attention was given to the actual care and treatment of patients. Success of treatment could be seen in the marked increase in the discharge rates of patients from hospital.

In the late 1920s insulin coma therapy was considered by many psychiatrists to be the treatment of choice for the patient with a well-established schizophrenic condition. The aim of treatment was to render a state of unconsciousness in the patient for approximately one hour each day. However, empirical studies in the 1950s showed that such treatment was no more effective than sleep induced by other drugs such as barbituates. The 1930s witnessed the introduction of the so-called shock-therapies. Based on the false belief that epilepsy was rare in schizophrenia, injections of chemicals such as cardiazal and camphor oil, and later the use of electric current, were employed to produce epileptic form fits in patients suffering from schizophrenia. Although crude, the results obtained, particularly later with depressed patients, were very encouraging. The mode of action of electro-convulsive therapy is still uncertain. Modified by the introduction of anaesthesia, muscle relaxants and pre-medication, it still remains a 'reserved' method of treatment in certain psychotic conditions. The 1930s saw also the introduction of psychosurgery. A Portuguese surgeon, Egas Moniz, performed the first pre-frontal leucotomy dividing the pathways between the frontal lobes and the thalamus. Based on observations of individuals suffering from injury to the frontal regions of the brain, pre-frontal leucotomy was used (with equivocal results) to treat a wide range of patients, including involutional melancholia and aggressive violent individuals. Alas, like the aforementioned treatments, pre-frontal leucotomy when 'successful' afforded only symptomatic relief and was of little value in effecting a cure.

At this time many criticisms were levelled at the earlier physical treatments. Butler and Rosenthall (1978) highlighted that many of these treatments were discovered almost by accident with no theoretical basis or understanding of why they worked. They added that many 'treatments', instead of being therapeutic, had in fact disastrous effects on some patients. Leucotomy, for example, when fashionable, was used indiscriminately, particularly on many chronic psychiatric patients. The legacy of such flagrant abuse of patients (perhaps for experimental purposes) can still be witnessed in many long-stay wards.

The 1940s and 1950s saw the introduction of the therapeutic community concept into psychiatry. Born out of experience gained in the treatment of demoralised soldiers after the second world war, Dr T. Main sought to create an environment wherein every single aspect of its structure and function, and the attitudes and behaviour of each one of its staff members, would be regarded as having a potentially therapeutic effect on the patient's care. Maxwell Jones, during the same period, developed the 'social model' of the therapeutic community which involved free communication and a lessening of the hierarchical effect. He suggested the necessity for the environment of the psychiatric hospital to be as similar as possible to the social organisation that exists in the community outside (see Jones, 1968, for a detailed description of the therapeutic community). In so doing Main, Jones and other therapeutic community exponents, helped introduce a social model of care into psychiatry. By enabling staff and patients to confront each other with their behaviour, the aim was to heighten self-awareness which would eventually lead to maturation and growth of the individual's personality. Although the concept may not have been widely accepted in its entirety, many of the therapeutic community principles are practised today, albeit in a diluted version.

In the 1950s another important milestone was reached in the treatment of mental disorder. The development of tranquillising drugs not only reduced the incidence of disturbed and violent behaviour, but also rendered the patient more amenable and approachable. The first of these, chlorpromazine, has been used widely since 1954 and has been followed by a variety of similar acting drugs. Unlike the overall dampening effect of sedatives, chlorpromazine works selectively on the emotional and motor functions, leaving thinking processes and memory largely unaffected. In so doing it causes no impairment in the level of awareness but reduces levels of inappropriate emotional and motor behaviour. Like many previous treatments, however, tranquillisers treat only the symptoms and fail to eradicate the cause. Since a withdrawal of medication frequently resulted in an exacerbation of the psychotic condition, long-term maintenance doses were often required. Because of the nature of schizophrenia, frequent relapses occurred due to the patient omitting medication. The advent of long-acting tranquillisers in the form of depot injections greatly helped to overcome this problem. The contribution of tranquillisers in the treatment of schizophrenia has been invaluable, not only affording speedy relief for patients in the acute phase but also enabling many chronic patients to leave hospital and live in the community.

Until recently, employment of patients was thought to be beneficial. Born out of the 'Protestant ethic' principle that mental imbalance rested on the fact that mental disturbance was the work of the devil and idleness opened the door for the devil, the working of patients in gardens, farms, wards and laundries was widely accepted. Allegations in the early 1960s that such work was cheap labour, saw the shift of emphasis to other forms of programmed activity. The development of different types of therapies, including recreational, occupational, social and industrial, brought with them a more individualised treatment regime. Although the assessment criterion used initially was rather primitive, attempts were at last being made to meet the individual needs of the patient instead of mass management.

The importance of psychiatric community care was highlighted in the 1959 Mental Health Act which recognised that the treatment of people suffering from psychiatric illness should be shifted as far as possible from institutional care to care within the community, and implied the setting up of a comprehensive psychiatric community care service. As well as being economically more viable (cheaper to keep patient in community than hospital), community care helped to alleviate the stigma and effects of institutionalisation associated with hospital care. Equally important, it allowed for the expansion of more social forms of treatment, directed at enabling the patient to cope more effectively in social situations.

The need to expand the psychiatric community care services was the result of many factors. Unquestionably, tranquillisers played a major role in affording the patient greater mental stability and preventing deterioration and relapse. The provision by local authorities of psychiatric units and day hospitals attached to general hospitals, sheltered workshops, housing and hostel accommodation not only assisted the patient to remain in the community, but also helped to educate the public by bridging the gap between mental hospitals and society. The transition from hospital to community care has, however, been slow. Promises by local authorities to make provision for the mentally ill in the community have received low priority. The DHSS document *Better Services for the Mentally Ill* (1975), perhaps in an attempt to placate growing unrest regarding the nature of services being provided, reiterated the importance of accommodating psychiatric patients outside large institutions. Alas, government finances to facilitate such a transition were not made available, resulting in many recommendations remaining unfulfilled.

Models of Care

Until the 1960s the treatment of psychiatric disorders was based primarily on the traditional 'medical model' emphasising that mental disorders are illnesses like any other illness. Using such a model a depressed patient, for example, could be considered as having some disturbance in the central nervous system or perhaps some biochemical abnormality that required the same principles of diagnosis, treatment and cure as any physical illness (see Figure 3.1).

In the late 1950s and early 1960s, however, greater recognition was given to a 'psychological model' of care in the form of behaviour therapy. Where Freud's psychological theory, in the form of psychoanalysis, highlighted the need to help patients achieve a better understanding of their feelings and motives so they could cope better with problems, studies including Wolpe (1958), Bandura (1969), and Lazarus (1971) emphasised treatment through a behaviourist approach called behaviour therapy or behaviour modification. Behaviour therapy focused not on patient insight, but on the problem behaviour itself. Based on the assumption that maladaptive behaviour in mentally ill patients is learned, behaviourists recommend that techniques developed in experimental work on learning can be employed to substitute new

Figure 3.1: Medical Model

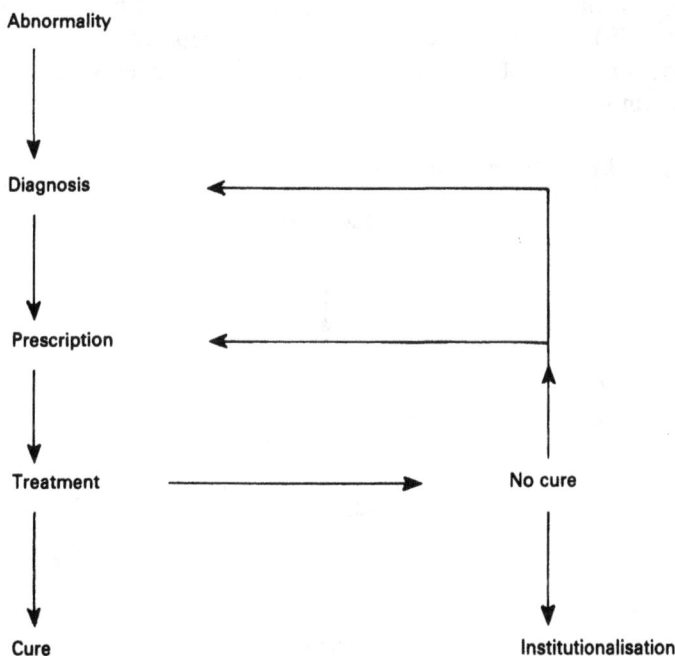

Abnormality

↓

Diagnosis

↓

Prescription

↓

Treatment ⟶ No cure

↓

Cure

Institutionalisation

and more appropriate responses for the maladaptive ones. Different behavioural techniques including systematic desensitisation and aversion therapy were introduced, with varying degrees of success, to treat conditions including phobias, obsessional states and alcohol dependence.

In addition to a medical and psychological model, there developed in the 1960s an interest in a social model of mental health care (see Figure 3.2). Exponents of the social model recognise that all people live in groups and that mental disorder arises when people can no longer, for various reasons (as discussed in Chapter 2), function properly within the group to which they belong. Their concern is with the roles assumed by people or assigned to them by others and how they behave within their roles. Social psychotherapeutic techniques including individual, group, marital and family therapy, developed during this era are now used widely throughout the psychiatric field to help emotionally disturbed individuals modify their behaviour so that they can adjust more satisfactorily to their social surroundings. Included also within this model of care SST, with its origins in behavioural psychology, linguistics and sociology, has been developed as a method of teaching the skills of social interaction in a systematic way. SST has been used with increasing popularity and success over a number of years with many psychiatric patients deficient in certain social skills.

Figure 3.2: Social Model

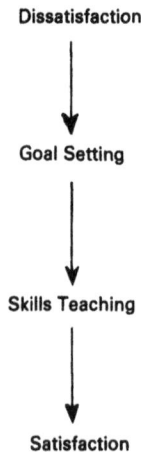

Dissatisfaction

↓

Goal Setting

↓

Skills Teaching

↓

Satisfaction

The development of a psychological and social model of care has seen correspondingly less emphasis placed on a medical doctrine. Nevertheless, to enable a patient to receive the greatest benefit from treatment, the relevance of all models should be considered.

In this historical review of psychiatry we have concentrated primarily upon changes effected from within (e.g. new schools of thought and methods of treatment). (For a comprehensive historical review of psychiatry see Foucault, 1979.) Cognisance, however, must also be taken of factors from without, such as sociological factors which help determine the treatment approach used. Although major tranquillisers and community care have resulted in a decline in the number of psychotic patients in hospital, manifestations of today's affluent society including stress and strain have led to correspondingly marked increases in conditions such as alcoholism, drug addiction and depression. While particular types of treatment (e.g. physical forms of treatment such as electro-convulsant therapy) may have been appropriate previously, evolving psychiatric disorders demand that treatments are also developed to meet the needs of today's society.

Evolution of Psychiatric Nursing

Bearing in mind this historical development of psychiatric care, the evolution of the psychiatric nurse's role will now be examined.

Psychiatric nursing has throughout the years been greatly influenced by the philosophy of treatment. Until the reforms of the last century, the predecessors of psychiatric nursing (keepers or attendants) provided primarily a custodial service with the responsibility of seeing that patients did not harm themselves or others, and ensuring that their basic bodily needs were attended to. They worked strictly under doctor's orders and were involved in such practices as purgation, beatings and physical restraint. One of the first to recognise the therapeutic potential of psychiatric nurses was Philippe Pinel in 1794. In his reforms he insisted on the necessity for kindness and understanding in the management of the mentally ill, and saw the personalities of both doctors and psychiatric nurses as the single most important factor in bringing about a cure. The role of the attendant Jean-Baptiste Pussin and his wife (an ex-patient) in Pinel's venture led to new responsibilities and emphases. Instead of merely providing custodial care they were actively involved in implementing and supporting Pinel's philosophy and played a vital part in the prevention of cruelty to patients and the institution of more humane methods of care. Later in 1856 Connelly, also recognising the importance of psychiatric nursing in treatment, stated 'the physician who understands the non-restraint system, well knows that attendants are his most essential instruments'.

Unfortunately, such revolutionary views were not universally accepted and custodial methods of treatment persisted right into the early twentieth century. A feature of custodial care during this era was the authority-submissive relationship between the nurse and patient. The criterion used by nursing staff to determine the efficiency of a ward or institution was often grossly misdirected. For example priorities such as tidiness, quietness and low expenditure were considered more important than the therapeutic atmosphere and quality of nurse-patient relationships. In order to meet these criteria psychiatric nurses were obliged to use their authority to gain patient submission and co-operation. The adoption of such criteria as highlighted by Martin (1974) was used to gain the approval of nursing administration. A ward that ran smoothly and viably was considered 'good', as were the staff who achieved it. Hence such requirements governed the role of the psychiatric nurse, resulting in work and discipline being more important than therapy. The remnants of such a philosophy can still be seen today in many long-stay wards.

Up until the mid-nineteenth century attendants were unqualified and completely subservient to the medical profession. With the development of county asylums, enlightened psychiatrists recognised the need for some form of training for the attendants. Hence a formal course of training was established by the Medico-Psychological Association (now the Royal College of Psychiatrists) in 1890, leading to the issue of nationally recognised certificates following examination. From 1891 the (Royal) Medico-Psychological Association was the main training and examining body for mental nurses until the General Nursing Council took over in 1951. There were initially problems in defining the actual role of the psychiatric nurse. As a result of uncertainty the objectives for training were medically orientated and were based on lectures in anatomy, physiology, hygiene, dietetics and basic nursing care. This, perhaps in the earlier part of this century, was sufficient as care was essentially medically determined. Physical treatments including electro-convulsive therapy, psychosurgery and insulin coma therapy required high degrees of clinical expertise and nursing care which qualified psychiatric nurses could offer. Although the 1930s and 1940s saw the first genuine attempts at treating patients, such treatments were nevertheless still employed within a custodial setting. This era also witnessed concomitant changes within the psychiatric nurse's role. Instead of being merely a passive bystander in the therapeutic arena, they were beginning to play an active role in the treatment process. Because of the uncompromising traditional environments in which such changes were taking place, however, the psychiatric nurse's primary function was still one of custodian.

The Psychiatric Nurse as a Therapeutic Agent

The radical changes in the 1950s and 1960s due largely to the advent of long-acting tranquillising drugs and the open-door policy, helped greatly to relegate the psychiatric nurse's custodial functions. Consequently the contribution of the nurse in the overall treatment programme was now being valued.

Warlingham Park Hospital and later Moorhaven in 1957 employed, for the first time, psychiatric nurses in the community despite opposition from social workers. The value of community psychiatric nurses is today fully recognised, and there can be few community areas in which the service has not been adopted. The progression from hospital to community, however, imposed new demands on the role of the psychiatric nurse. The constraints of institutions coupled with inadequate training schemes, ill-prepared nurses for working effectively within the patient's own home setting. Previously governed by medical staff, nurses were now being afforded autonomy and required to work as independent practitioners. Such radical developments necessitated a growth in the nurse's knowledge base. Previously concerned with physical and psychological aspects of care, cognisance was now taken of the sociological effects on mental health, including the role of the family and patient in treatment, the role of the patient within the family, and the effects of economics, work and leisure on health. To facilitate this change courses by the Joint Board of Clinical Nursing Studies (now embodied in the United Kingdom Central Council for Nurses, Midwives and Health Visitors) were designed to equip the nurse with the necessary theory and expertise.

The evolving emphasis placed on psychological and social models of health care during the 1950s and 1960s also necessitated the psychiatric nurse to take up new and varied roles within the hospital setting. Sabshin (1957), Maloney (1962) and later Trick and Obcarskas (1968) all highlighted the growing multi-dimensional nature of the role, including that of psychotherapist, technician and manager. The change of emphasis in the treatment philosophy helped identify the gross inadequacies of the then psychiatric nursing training syllabus. As a result, a new experimental training scheme was introduced in 1957 and officially adopted in 1964. With the inclusion of psychology, psychiatry and ward teaching in the new curriculum, students were afforded greater insight into both patients' conditions and the role of the nurse as therapeutic agent.

The 1960s and 1970s saw consolidation of the psychiatric nurse's generic role in treatment programmes. As greater emphasis was placed on psychological and social models of care, it became increasingly customary to see nurses involved in areas previously not considered their responsibility. A significant increase, for example, in alcohol and drug addiction saw a notable upsurge in group therapy in which nurses played an active part.

Until the 1970s the diversification of the nurse's role was greatly influenced from without. Although factors including behaviour therapy, therapeutic community, community care and societal changes undoubtedly played a part in moulding the psychiatric nurse's role, there was an increasing need to develop professional identity. Such a quest over recent years, perhaps as a result of the inability to define with precision the term psychiatric nursing, has resulted in much introspection and constructive criticism, leading to the recognition of the need for a psychiatric nursing model of care. Such a model of care, based on the 'nursing process', has been fervently expounded over the past few years and has been inculcated into the new psychiatric nursing syllabus. By adopting a 'nursing model of care' it is hoped that task-orientated procedures will be replaced by care tailored to meet the individual needs of the patients. By so doing, Dickinson (1982) claims nurses will become independent and expert practitioners whose authority is based upon nursing knowledge. She believes this will undoubtedly bring nursing closer to the professional trait model.

Specialisation in Psychiatric Nursing

While the 1960s and 1970s saw a dramatic development in the psychiatric nurse's responsibilities, there has in the 1980s been mounting pressure to move from a generic role to specialisation. The specialist role of the nurse in the general setting has been widely recognised and accepted. The pursuit of specialisation within psychiatric nursing, however, is only now gathering momentum. As far back as 1968 the Ministry of Health encouraged the view that expansions in the clinical roles of psychiatric nurses should be made, recommending that there should be 'experimental courses at basic and higher levels with a view to preparing nurses for an advanced clinical role'. By specialising, they claimed, psychiatric nurses would gain a more thorough understanding of the sociological and psychological implications of caring for the mentally ill. Both the Briggs Report (DHSS, 1972) and later the United Central Council (UKCC) consultation document on education and training, suggested similar provisions, stating that psychiatric nurses should be given the opportunity to specialise following qualification. The Royal College of Psychiatrists (1973) reiterated the need to move from the generic role when in the Tait Report they stated 'We are disappointed that the nursing profession has not, as yet, brought forward positive proposals which would remedy the present deficiencies of numbers, quality and *specialism.*'

Specialisation has nevertheless taken place. Many, for example, believe community psychiatric nursing to be a speciality, although when critically analysed there is evidence to suggest that their training and clinical expertise is still primarily generic in nature. However, practising clinical nurse specialists do exist. In recent years, increasing attention has been paid to the development of a nurse role that has as its prime objective the therapeutic modification of patients' behaviour. Marks et al (1975) concluded that nurse therapists in behaviour therapy 'treated phobic patients as successfully as psychiatrists and psychologists using similar psychological treatments in comparable psychiatric populations'. In ascertaining the effectiveness of nurse therapists in behaviour therapy, Bird et al (1979) concluded that the results of such studies indicated that the potential value of psychiatric nurses warranted further development.

Psychiatric nurses using specialist clinical expertise in several other areas have also been carefully scrutinised with promising results. Examples are the nurse as surrogate junior psychiatrist on long-stay wards (Whitehead and Fannon, 1971), as preliminary decision maker in general practice (Moore et al 1973), and as co-practitioner in primary care (Scherer et al 1977). The role of the psychiatric nurse in SST has, in particular, received much interest in recent years, as part of both a generic and specialist role. The Briggs Report (DHSS, 1972) and more recently the Mental Nurse training syllabus (National Board for Nursing, Midwifery, and Health Visiting, 1983) both identified the need for nurses to be familiar with social methods of treatment. This is reflected in the new training schemes currently being implemented.

Specialisation in SST.   Pressures are mounting on nurses to specialise in SST. Firstly, by adopting a nursing model of care, psychiatric nurses now have, in the shape of the nursing process, a framework similar to that used in SST (see Chapter 5):

(1) Assessment: of social skills deficits
(2) Planning: selection of targets etc
(3) Implementation: SST strategy employed — instruction/modelling etc
(4) Evaluation: through feedback/discussion/video playback etc.

With the basic frameworks of care being alike, psychiatric nurses can adapt more readily to SST techniques.

Secondly, as highlighted by Trower et al (1978) 'A good therapeutic relationship is an important pre-requisite in SST, initially to help the patient understand his problem and accept training and subsequently to increase the therapist's effectiveness as a model and reinforcer'. The therapeutic effectiveness of the nurse-patient relationship has been widely recognised and studied. Ferguson and Carney (1970), for example, from their studies found that patients were of the opinion that their 'relationships' with nurses were of more therapeutic benefit than were their 'relationships' with doctors and social workers. Others, including Altschul (1964) and O'Hare (1972), have suggested that the prime quality of a psychiatric nurse is an ability to form good relationships with others. Bearing in mind the importance of the trainer-patient relationship in SST programmes, psychiatric nurses have the necessary inter-personal attributes upon which SST success is determined.

Thirdly, there is increasing demand for social methods of treatment. As highlighted in Chapter 2, a great majority of psychiatric patients experience social skill difficulties, and this has led to the increased use of SST techniques as part of the overall treatment programme. Such an approach, however, requires both intensive and extensive individual attention, and special skills. The demand, as highlighted by Russell (1973) has unfortunately now outstripped supply. Fourthly, greater emphasis is now being placed on a multi-discipline approach to treatment. The range of issues in which it is accepted that a particular discipline's view must, by definition, take priority is increasingly narrow. Disciplines of many kinds, including psychiatric nurses, now expect a greater say in patient management.

Fifthly, although this is perhaps a less desirable reason for SST specialisation, due to economic constraints governments are naturally interested in using nursing staff to satisfy the demand for therapists. Finally, as argued by Peck (1973), nurses are already acting as agents of behavioural change but there is need for training so that they can carry it out more efficiently. Specialisation, therefore, by the psychiatric nurse in SST, may be seen merely as an extension of the existing generic role.

Overview

In this chapter the evolving role of the psychiatric nurse has been discussed. Because of the many changes in attitudes and approaches to mental health and illness in recent years, psychiatric nursing is in a period of transition. It is no longer professionally or morally acceptable for the nurse to merely give custodial care to the hospitalised patient. Nursing care is expected to be therapeutic, individualised and comprehensive. Such care requires *specialised* knowledge and understanding of human behaviour and greater specialist ability and skill in human relationships on the part of psychiatric nurses. As a result, the role of the psychiatric nurse should encompass that of social skills trainer. The nurse should, therefore, be familiar with the development and origins of SST, should be aware of the central tenets of this training method, and should be able to assist in the design, implementation and evaluation of SST programmes for specific groups of patients.

4 A MODEL OF INTERPERSONAL INTERACTION

In this chapter we examine a theoretical framework that can be applied to the analysis of interpersonal communication. In particular, this framework represents the theoretical underpinning for the social skills approach, since it is based upon the thesis that communication can be viewed in terms of skilled performance. As discussed in Chapter 1, this perspective developed from the initial investigations by psychologists into charting the nature and form of motor skills. It was the attempts to apply this knowledge directly to the analysis of social interaction that resulted in the eventual emergence of SST.

This chapter, therefore, is concerned with an analysis of the extent to which a theoretical model, developed for the study of motor skill, can be applied to the study of social skill. As such, it incorporates an examination of the central processes involved in skilled behaviour *per se*. Differences between motor and social skill are highlighted, and an extended model of interpersonal interaction is presented in order to account for those features that are peculiar to social encounters.

The Motor Skill Model

Although different theorists have postulated different types of model of motor skills, the central components of these models have certain commonalities. In particular, the skilled individual is conceived as carrying out a response, perceiving the outcome of this response and then making decisions about the next response. This can be exemplified with reference to the motor skill model put forward by Welford (1965). As outlined in Figure 4.1, Welford's model portrays the individual as perceiving information via the sense organs (ears, eyes, hands, nose etc.). A number of such perceptions are received and banked in the short-term memory store until sufficient data has been accumulated to enable a decision to be made about an appropriate response. This decision is facilitated by information retained in the long-term memory store. Once a decision has been made, a response is then

Figure 4.1: Welford's Model of the Human Sensory-motor System

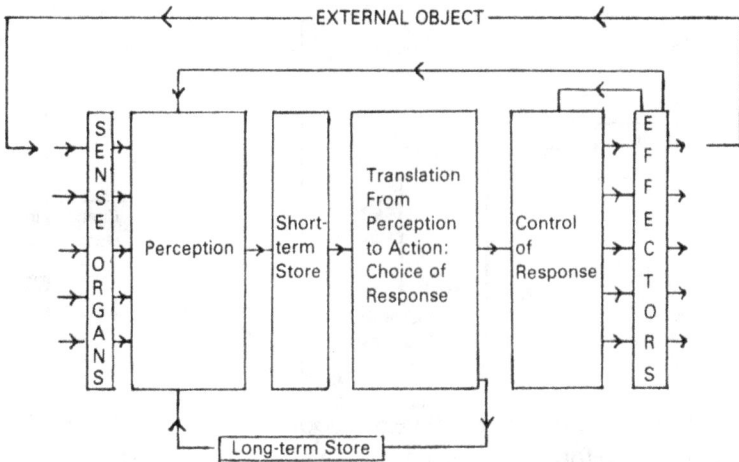

executed by the effector system (vocal organs, hands, head etc.). The outcome of this response is, in turn, monitored by the perceptual system, and so the process continues.

Thus, a car driver, attempting to park between two other cars, must consider factors such as the actual space between the two cars, the distance to leave in order to allow him to drive into the available space, and the extent to which he needs to turn the driving wheel to cut neatly into this space. All these details will be held in the short-term memory store, and compared with information from long-term memory regarding the width of his own vehicle and his previous experience of car parking. Using all this information, the driver will then respond by attempting to park his car. The success of his effort will be monitored and, where appropriate, stored in long-term memory to guide future behaviour in similar situations.

As this example illustrates, Welford's model does seem to account for the main processes involved in the performance of motor skills. However, Argyle and Kendon (1967) in arguing that there were many similarities between motor and social skills, modified this model slightly and applied it directly to the analysis of social performance. As Figure 4.2 illustrates, Argyle and Kendon simplified Welford's model by removing the memory store blocks, combining sense organs and perception, control of responses and

Figure 4.2: Argyle and Kendon's Motor Skill Model

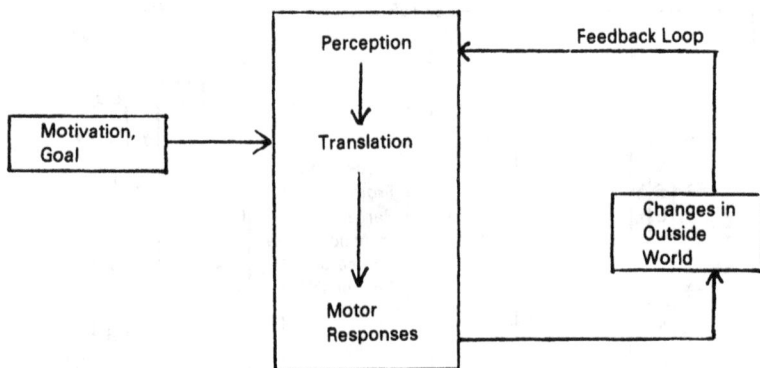

effectors, and adding the dimensions of motivation and goal. In essence, therefore, these two models are very similar. An example of how Argyle and Kendon's model can be applied to a social situation is confrontation by an overtly aggressive individual who is threatening violence against us. In such a situation we will want to avoid being physically harmed and so will be *motivated* to take some form of action. Our *goal* may then be to try to calm the person down. To do so we can *translate* various plans of action (say nothing, look concerned, say you are sorry about whatever has made him angry, burst into tears etc.), and *respond* by carrying out one of these plans. Following this response, we will monitor how the other person reacts (change in the outside world), and *perceive* this reaction, thereby enabling a decision to be made about the next response to make.

At a general level, it would therefore appear that social performance can be analysed in terms of a motor skill model, and that the same processes are involved in both motor and social skills. While this is partially true, it should also be realised that there are a number of important differences between these two sets of skills including the following:

(1) Social skills, by definition, necessitate the presence of another person with whom one is interacting, whereas many motor skills do not. One can walk, operate a machine, or have a swim, all of which involve motor skills, without other people being involved. In social interaction, however, we must con-

sider the goals and motivation of the other person, as well as our own. Thus, we judge the behaviour of others by what we consider their goals and motives to be. For example, if we know that someone has recently been bereaved, we would view their lack of interest in us as being due to the fact that they are grieving, rather than assuming that they just do not like us.

(2) Feelings and emotions are of vital import in social interaction. Our own feelings and emotional state will influence our behaviour, and, similarly, we are often concerned about the feelings of other people.

(3) The process of person perception differs in several respects from the perception of inanimate objects. Firstly, we perceive our own responses (we hear what we say and how we say it, and may be aware of our nonverbal behaviour) and use this information to judge our social performance. Secondly, we perceive the responses of others, and how they are responding to us. Thirdly, there is the aspect of metaperception which refers to the process whereby we attempt to decipher how the other person is perceiving us.

(4) Situational factors are important in inter-personal encounters. The nature of the task, the environment, the roles of the people involved and their cultural background will all have a bearing upon the behaviour of the interactors.

(5) Personal factors such as age, sex, and appearance will also influence the behaviour of people. Thus, we tend to stand further away from, and look less at, people with facial disfigurements, while standing closer to, and looking more at, attractive individuals.

Any model of social interaction must take account of these five features, and in Figure 4.3 we present an extension of Argyle and Kendon's model, in which we have attempted to cater for the specific features of social skill. This extended model represents both participants as having their own goals and motives. The term 'mediating factors' has been employed in order to take into consideration the emotional facets of human communication. Perception is portrayed as emanating from both one's own responses and those of the other person. Finally, personal and situational factors are recognised as impinging upon the whole interactive process. Taking this model as a basis for understanding social

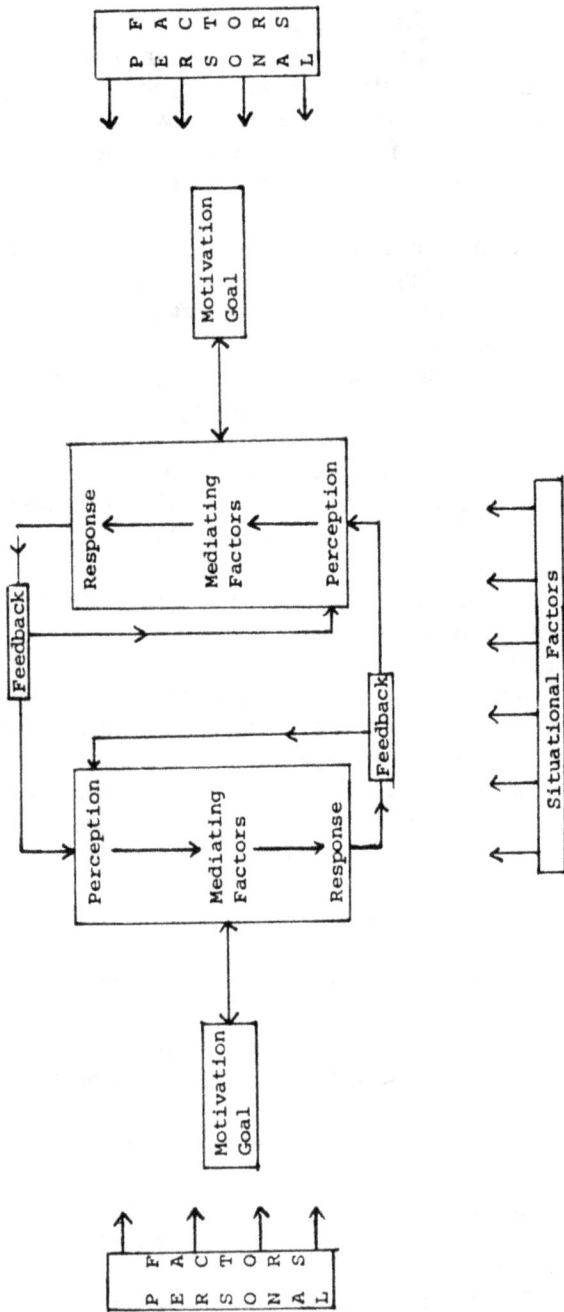

Figure 4.3: Extended Model of Interpersonal Interaction

interaction, we will now examine each of the elements within the model.

Goals and Motivation

The starting point for this extended model of interpersonal inter-action is the goals being pursued by the individuals, and the degree of motivation that they have to achieve these. Motivation is, in turn, directly influenced by needs. There are a large number of human needs that have to be satisfied to enable us to live our lives to the fullest possible extent. Some of these needs are more important than others, and different psychologists have proposed differing theories about the nature of human needs. One of the best known of these is the hierarchy of human needs devised by Ibrahim Maslow (1954), as exemplified in Figure 4.4.

As Maslow's hierarchy illustrates, the most important needs are physiological, being concerned with the survival of the individual. Thus, if we are very hungry, thirsty or cold, we will be very highly motivated to rectify this deprivation, and our goal will be to seek food, water or heat. If these needs have been satisfied we will then be concerned with the next level, namely safety needs such as security and freedom from fear. We meet these needs by a whole range of methods including locking our doors at night, establishing

Figure 4.4: Maslow's Hierarchy of Human Needs

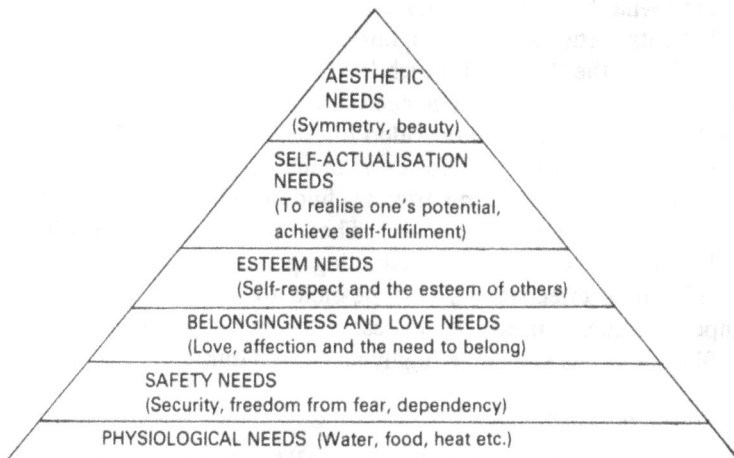

police forces, saving our money 'for a rainy day'. Once these needs have been met, we then become concerned with belonging and love needs, such as the need to be loved or accepted and not to be lonely or isolated. Making friends, getting married, or joining a club are all means whereby we attempt to cater for this type of need. At the next level are the esteem needs, which can be satisfied in a number of ways including occupational status or achievement in some other sphere. At a higher level is the need for self-actualisation, which is concerned with realising one's full potential. People continually seek new challenges and undertake various apparently pointless exercises to meet this need (e.g. running marathons, climbing mountains).

Once all of the above needs have been satisfied, the individual may then become concerned with aesthetic needs, such as the pursuit of beauty by purchasing rare paintings, having cosmetic surgery, or wearing exquisite jewellery. Maslow argues that only when the lower needs are met will we seek to satisfy higher needs. The person who is suffering from hunger will usually seek food at all costs, even risking personal security, and will beg, if necessary, without concern for self-esteem. Equally, someone in a secure, well-paid salaried job, may resign and proceed to open their own business in order to attempt to become 'self-actualised'. However, while this hierarchy is valid for most instances of human needs, there are exceptions, and needs can be influenced directly by goals. One example of this occurs when political prisoners forego physiological needs by starving themselves to death in order to achieve what they regard as higher-order goals.

Patients participating in programmes of SST will usually be concerned with the third and fourth levels of need, namely belonging and love needs, and esteem needs. In our society, the first two levels of need are usually provided for, in that few of us will starve to death or die violently. However, many people find difficulty in meeting strangers, making friends, finding a partner and being assertive and respected by others. These are the facets with which SST is concerned, and by facilitating patients to improve their interpersonal effectiveness it is possible to help them to satisfy important human needs. By the same token, patients who wish to fulfil these needs should be highly motivated during SST.

Theories of Motivation

Three main theories of motivation have been postulated. The

earliest of these is 'drive theory' which regards humans as being motivated by drives, which are in turn activated by needs. So, when we are hungry we have a drive to behave in such a fashion as to obtain food, when thirsty we are driven to seek a drink and so on. When the goal of the drive has been attained, drive reduction is said to have occurred, and this results in a pleasant internal state. Although this theory can obviously be applied to a great deal of human behaviour, it does not satisfactorily account for many behaviours such as climbing a dangerous mountain, hang gliding or going on frightening rides in an amusement park. In all of these instances drives would be increased rather than decreased. Furthermore, drive theory fails to take account of the effects of external stimuli on human behaviour. Someone who is not initially hungry may be tempted to eat by the sight of cakes in a cafe window. In this case the cakes can be viewed as an incentive to eat.

This explanation forms the basis of a second theory of motivation, namely 'incentive theory', which emphasises the importance of external incentives as motivation for behaviour. A central tenet of this theory is that we seek positive incentives and avoid negative incentives. If we are hungry, food will be a positive incentive and approached, whereas the sight of a bully at school would be a negative incentive and avoided. In both of these cases the incentives are clearly positive or negative, but where an incentive has both positive and negative aspects, anxiety may result. In laboratory experiments, hungry animals who have to undergo an electric shock in order to secure food display varying levels of distress or anxiety, depending upon the strength of the shock. This process has been termed 'approach/avoidance conflict'. A similar process can be observed in humans. A selection interview is a tense situation for most people, yet one that can result in a positive outcome, and so candidates will usually display anxiety before such interviews. Similarly, social inadequates will find many interactive situations distressing, yet may wish to engage in them in order to make friends or overcome loneliness. SST, by increasing their confidence and ability, can serve to decrease the negative incentives of such situations.

Arousal is an important aspect of both drive (where it is seen as being due to deprivation) and incentive (where it is viewed as the result of external stimuli) theories. A recognition of the crucial role of arousal has led to the third theory of motivation, 'arousal theory', wherein motivation is regarded as being one among a number of causes of arousal (other causes include novel events, environmental factors such as noise or other people and drugs). Level of arousal has a direct effect upon performance, in that if we are either over-aroused or under-aroused, our performance will be adversely affected. Arousal levels vary from one person to another. Some people need a lot of stimulation and become bored easily, whereas others prefer a minimum of stimulation and become disturbed if the level of stimulation is too high. Those with low levels of arousal prefer safe, quiet environments, whereas those with high levels are more effective in challenging, changing situations. Individuals need to be aware of their arousal threshold in order to select contexts in which they will perform effectively.

Goals and Behaviour

Motivation is therefore important in determining the goals that we seek, and these goals will have a direct influence upon our behaviour. We interpret the behaviour of others based upon the goals that they are pursuing, although we are not always accurate in these interpretations. People can deceive us in terms of their true goals, so that someone may be friendly towards us for reasons other than their liking for us. However, our judgements about the goals of others, based upon their behaviour, are often accurate, and because of this we are shocked when someone whom we trusted as having honourable goals turns out to have hidden goals. Furthermore, judgements about the goals of behaviour can be of crucial importance, as when a courtroom jury has to decide whether a killing by a defendant was accidental or premeditated.

Behaviour can be guided either by conscious or subconscious goals. In the former case, the individual will be aware of his behaviour and of the reasons why for it, will have planned it and will be able to explain and justify it in relation to the underlying goal. Often, however, we operate at a more subconscious level in terms of goals. Indeed, this is a feature of skilled behaviour, in that the experienced interviewer will ask questions, provide reward etc. without consciously thinking about so doing, just as the experienced driver will turn on the ignition, engage gear etc. without being consciously aware of the goals of the behaviour. An important dimension of skilled behaviour is this capacity to act and react quickly at a subconscious level (see Chapter 1 for a further analysis of the nature of skill).

A distinction also needs to be made between long-term and

short-term goals. Our behaviour is guided by short-term goals, with long-term goals being achieved through a sub-set of short-term ones. In order to make friends we have to meet people, open a conversation, provide reward, look for common areas of interest and so on. If these short-term goals are not met, then the long-term one of making friends will not be attained. However, on occasions, goal conflict may occur where the short-term and long-term goals may not concur. Telling a good friend that he has an annoying habit, while maintaining the same level of friendship, would be an example of conflicting goals. Encounters such as this obviously require great skill and tact, and will be difficult for most patients involved in SST.

Some patients will also have inappropriate goals or expectancies in a given situation. For example, they may see a selection interviewer as someone who will give them careers guidance. Another problem at this stage is that some patients may feel that they have no clear goals to pursue, as with depressed patients who feel they have nothing to live for. This may be the result of repeated failure in social interaction, which eventually leads to a withdrawal from such interactions. With these patients, building up a meaningful, and attainable, goal structure is an important step in remediation.

Goals, therefore, play a vital role in determining behaviour. Once appropriate goals have been decided upon, these will influence the way we perceive others, interpret situations and respond. The next stage of the model is the phase involving mediating factors.

Mediating Factors

Mediating factors are those internal states, activities or processes within the individual which mediate between the goal being pursued, the feedback perceived, and the response made. These factors influence the way people and events are perceived, and determine the capacity of the individual to assimilate, process and respond to the social information received during inter-personal encounters. At this stage, the individual makes decisions about the likelihood of goals being achieved, and decides upon an appropriate course of action. We will focus upon two main mediating factors, namely cognition and emotion.

Cognition

Cognition has been defined as 'all the processes by which the sensory input is transformed, reduced, elaborated, stored, recovered and used' (Neisser, 1967). This definition encapsulates the central aspects of cognition. This involves *transforming*, or decoding and making sense of the sensory information that is perceived. To do so it is often necessary to *reduce* the amount of information attended to in order to avoid over-loading the system. Conversely, at times it is necessary to *elaborate* upon minimal information by making interpretations, judgements or evaluations (e.g. if someone refuses to speak to us, we will attempt to work out why this is so). Some of the incoming information will be stored in either the short-term or the long-term memory. Short-term memory involves the retention of information for a few minutes, while long-term memory refers to retention over weeks, months or years. Information stored in short-term memory will quickly be lost unless it is transferred to the long-term store, where it becomes resistant to loss. Thus, elderly patients may vividly remember aspects of their childhood, yet be unable to retain recent information.

One theory that has been put forward to account for memory is that we use a process known as 'context-dependent coding', wherein remembering occurs by recalling the context of the original event. When we meet someone we recognise but cannot place, we try to think of when and where we encountered them before — in other words, we try to put them in a particular context. A similar process occurs during social interaction, whereby we evaluate people and situations in terms of our experience of previous similar encounters. In this way we recover or retrieve information that is stored, to facilitate the processes of decision making and problem solving, with existing circumstances being related to previous knowledge and experience. Cognitions therefore play an important role in skilled performance.

Socially skilled individuals will have greater control over their thought processes and will use these to monitor and regulate their behaviour in relation to the responses of others. This meshing of responses necessitates an awareness of the ability level of the other person, and of the 'way they think', since 'in order to interact successfully and repeatedly with the same persons, one must have the capacity to form cognitive conceptions of the others' cognitive conceptions' (Wessler, 1984). The person high in social skill will have an ability to size up people and situations more rapidly and respond more appropriately than the person who is low in social skill.

As Shaw (1979) points out, however, some thinking and remembering is purposeful and goal-oriented while other mental activity is less controlled and has an automatic, involuntary nature. The extent to which these automatic thoughts interrupt the main direction of mental activity varies from person to person, but is characteristic of many patients, such as schizophrenics, in whom a large number of unrelated thoughts 'flood through' the mind. This results in a poor capacity to process incoming information logically, coupled with misinterpretation of this information. Depressed or anxious patients often suffer from negative thoughts and irrational beliefs. It has also been found that depressed people tend to suffer from memory distortion in that they tend to distort their memories of events in a negative direction (by emphasising the bad experiences) whereas normal people distort their memories in a positive direction (by remembering the better features). Where extreme distortions of cognition occur, SST will not usually be a suitable method of treatment, since this method involves patient awareness of the goals of training and commitment to the training programme (see Chapter 5). With many patients, however, this method will be suitable and, as Curran et al (1984) point out, will 'be particularly helpful in facilitating the acquisition of new cognitions', by encouraging patients to develop techniques for coping with various social situations.

Emotion

There are three main components of emotion. Firstly, the direct conscious experience or feeling of emotion; secondly, the physiological processes that accompany emotions; and, thirdly, the observable actions used to signal and express emotions. In noting the importance of emotions, Izard (1977) states, 'virtually all of the neurophysiological systems and subsystems of the body are involved in greater or lesser degree in emotional states. Such changes inevitably affect the perceptions, thoughts and actions of the person'. Thus, a depressed person will tend to focus upon negative cues, adopt a slouched posture and flat tone of voice and generally avoid interacting with others, whereas a happy person will pick up positive cues and display signs of happiness by smiling, being lively and joining in social interaction.

The exact nature of the relationship between cognitions and emotions is, however, unclear. Some theorists argue that a direct causal relationship exists in that emotions are controlled by cognitions. Within this model, irrational beliefs would be seen as causing fear or anxiety, which could in turn be remedied by helping the individual to become more rational about his or her beliefs. This perspective is regarded by other theorists as being an over-simplication of the relationship between thought and affect. It is argued that emotional states can also cause changes in cognition, so that an individual who is very angry may not be able to 'think straight' while it is also possible to be 'out of your mind' with worry. It therefore appears that a reciprocal relationship exists between cognitions and emotions, in that the way we think can influence how we feel and vice versa.

Emotional states are therefore very important in relation to the goals we pursue, how we interpret the responses of others and the way in which we react. One indicator of the importance of emotions is the fact that we have a large number of labels that we use to describe various emotional experiences. Averill (1975) carried out a study in which he identified a total of 558 discrete terms for emotions. While some of these emotions appear to be expressed in a common fashion across cultures (interest, joy, surprise, distress, disgust, anger, shame and fear) there are also differences between cultures in the display and acceptability of emotion (e.g. 'inscrutable' Japanese and 'expressive' Italians).

Emotional disorder is a function of most types of psychiatric patient. Schizophrenics often report that they have no feelings or that they feel empty, and this is reflected in a typical dull, flat facial expression, sometimes referred to as 'flattened affect'. Similarly, extremes of emotion can be found amongst patients suffering from, for example, anxiety, depression or paranoia. Since SST is likely to induce anxiety in even the most stable of individuals, patients need to be selected carefully and monitored constantly during training, to ensure that they do not suffer from undue stress.

While emotion and cognition are the two main aspects that we have focused upon, other mediating factors have a bearing on the way we process information. Our values and beliefs will influence our perceptions, actions, cognitions and emotions. Thus, a racist will tend to behave in a certain way towards members of another race who are viewed as inferior. At a more subtle level we can be influenced by the accent of others into behaving in certain ways (e.g. people with 'posh' accents are usually treated with respect, being viewed as intelligent). Values and beliefs can, therefore, influence our attitudes to others. Attitudes are also affected by our previous experiences of the person with whom we are interacting and by our experiences of similar people. Finally, the disposition of the individual is an important facet in determining responses in any given situation. Factors such as whether the person is shy, out-going, competitive, co-operative, aggressive or submissive will influence both how situations are perceived and what types of response are carried out.

All these mediating factors come together at the decision making stage, before a response is initiated in social interaction. This process, of translating perceptions into actions, will take place at a subconscious level if the performance is skilled. At the stage of skill learning such translations may be conscious. The learner driver will think about changing gear, turning the steering wheel, indicating, etc., but when he or she becomes skilled such actions are carried out automatically. A similar process occurs during SST, when patients are made aware of, and taught to think about, what they are doing during social interaction. This can interfere with the communication process itself (similar to the 'kangaroo petrol' syndrome among learner drivers), and it is only once their actions become subconscious again that improvements in skill can be evaluated. Patients may therefore need assurance that any inter-ference is a temporary phenomenon, and will be beneficial in the long-term. This phenomenon of 'training dips' is also common in the coaching of various sports, where the athlete's performance can deteriorate slightly during training, but will improve after the training programme.

Responses

When a goal has been formulated and a plan of action decided upon, the next step is to implement this plan by carrying out a social response. It is the function of the response system (voice, hands, face etc.) to implement the plan by employing a range of behaviours. Judgements about social skill are based upon the response capacity of the individual. If someone is able to describe appropriate behaviour in any given social situation, but cannot put this behaviour into practice, we would say that they are not socially skilled. It is the ability to perform effectively which is one of the defining features of skilled behaviour. In fact, the skilled performer may find it difficult to verbalise or explain their behaviour. Thus, the skilled footballer may be unable to provide a loquacious rationale for his performance ('I hit it and it went in'), whereas the commentator who can explain in depth how and why the footballer succeeded will often be unable to display any actual footballing skills himself. In SST, therefore, it is of crucial importance that the patient learns to use social skills appropriately. For this reason, practicals play a vital role in this type of training (see Chapter 5).

Social behaviour can be categorised into a number of component areas. As Figure 4.5 indicates, an initial distinction can be made between linguistic and non-linguistic behaviour. Linguistic behaviour encompasses all aspects associated with the spoken word, including the actual verbal content (the words we use), and the paralinguistic messages associated with it. Paralanguage refers to the way in which something is said as opposed to what is said, and includes the pitch, tone, speed, volume, and accent of the voice, as well as pauses, interruptions and speech dysfluencies. Non-linguistic behaviour involves all of our bodily communication and is concerned with the study of what we do rather than what we say. It can be subdivided into three main dimensions. 'Tacesics' is the systematic study of body contact; 'proxemics' is the systematic study of the spatial features of social presentation (interpersonal distance, orientation, territoriality etc.); and kinesics is the systematic study of body motion (facial expressions, head movements, posture, gestures, gaze etc.) (Scherer and Ekman, 1982).

The central thrust of SST is to provide the patient with an analysis of social responses in such a way that these responses can be learned. This necessitates reducing interpersonal interaction

Figure 4.5: Classifications of Social Behaviour

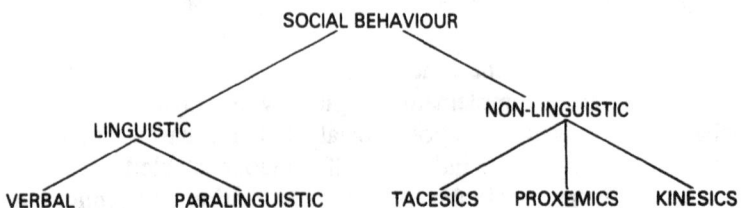

SOCIAL BEHAVIOUR

LINGUISTIC   NON-LINGUISTIC

VERBAL   PARALINGUISTIC   TACESICS   PROXEMICS   KINESICS

into smaller identifiable sequences, or units, of behaviour, and allowing the patient to practise each unit separately. The nurse must therefore be familiar with the range of social behaviours that have been identified, and be aware of how these behaviours interrelate (see Chapters 7, 8 and 9). It should be remembered that skilled behaviour is hierarchically organised with larger tasks comprising smaller component units. An example of this is given by McFall (1982) in relation to the task of finding a spouse:

> Nested within that global task would be smaller tasks, like 'meeting potential spouses', 'dating', and 'developing an intimate relationship'. Dating, in turn, might be broken into sub-tasks, such an initiating, conversing, parting etc. Each of these could be sub-divided further into component tasks, for example, initiating a date might be segmented into smaller task units such as selecting a person to approach, arranging for an opportunity to make the overture, and proposing the date. Conceivably, each of these might be decomposed into even smaller units.

This type of analysis can be applied to the types of situation that patients undergoing SST may find difficult, thereby identifying for each situation a hierarchy of tasks and skills which can be studied sequentially.

Learning

As discussed in Chapter 1, social behaviour is learned through a process of modelling and imitation of significant others. This begins at an early age and, as Bandura (1967) points out:

> The pervasiveness of this form of learning is clearly evident in naturalistic observations of children's play in which they frequently reproduce the entire parental role, including the appropriate mannerisms vocal inflections and attitudes, much to the parents' surprise and embarrassment.

As the child develops, he or she will then use significant others for behaviour models, including peers, pop stars, film actors or sports personalities. The greater the range of effective models available, the greater the likelihood will be that the child will acquire effective social behaviours.

Family and class background have been found to have a marked effect on the use of language. Bernstein (1971) made a distinction between two language codes, a restricted code which is used primarily by the working class (unskilled and semi-skilled workers), and an elaborated code used predominantly by the 'middle class'. The main differences between the two codes are that compared with the elaborated code the restricted code involves:

(1) Shorter and simpler sentences
(2) A more limited vocabulary with frequent use of traditional, idiomatic expressions
(3) Greater use of personal pronouns (I, we, you) as opposed to impersonal pronouns (one, it)
(4) Repetitive use of conjunctions (because, so, then, but)
(5) 'Sympathetic circularity', which involves the use of statements phrased as questions ('... know what I mean?' '... you know?' '... isn't it?')
(6) Increased tendency to replace reason by command. Bernstein (1961) exemplifies this with reference to a mother-child interaction on a bus, beginning wih the working class example:
Mother Hold on tight
Child Why?
Mother You'll fall
Child Why?
Mother I told you to hold on tight, didn't I?'

and contrasting this with the middle class example:

Mother Hold on tight
Child Why?
Mother If you don't you will be thrown forward and you'll fall
Child Why?
Mother Because if the bus suddenly stops you'll jerk forward on to the seat in front.

These examples are illustrative of two different types of model. Individuals receiving the second type of model will be more likely to have acquired greater linguistic ability. Modelling is, therefore, an important aspect in the learning of social skills, and the nurse should provide patients with appropriate models during SST. (This aspect is explored in Chapter 5.) The use of these models will be dependent upon the type of skill deficit displayed by the patient. Lack of social skill may be due to three main causes:

(1) The patient has not learned appropriate social behaviours. In this instance the primary task will be to enable the patient to acquire those social skills in which he or she is deficient

(2) The patient demonstrates a lack of skill in specific contexts. Thus, a male may be able to converse with other males, but may find extreme difficulty in interacting with females. The focus here will be upon the application of skills that the patient already has, to specific situations

(3) The patient has learned the skilled behaviours but uses them inappropriately by, for example, asking personal questions to complete strangers, staring at others, or laughing at the wrong moment. In other words, the patient says or does the right thing at the wrong time. Here, the focus will be upon encouraging the patient to control his or her skills more effectively.

Learning to use social responses effectively is the main objective of SST for patients. Not only should they learn to recognise a range of important inter-personal behaviours, but they should also be given the opportunity to practise these in the controlled training environment. In this way, the patient's repertoire of social skills can be developed and refined.

Feedback and Perception

Once a response has been carried out, feedback is available to the individual. Feedback enables the person to evaluate the effectiveness of responses and alter subsequent behaviour accordingly. In order to perform any task it is necessary to receive such feedback, in terms of 'knowledge of results' of the performance (Annett, 1969). We need to know how effective or ineffective our initial performance has been, in order to take corrective action where necessary. We could not effectively drive a car, throw darts or even walk along a straight line if we were unable to see the results of our actions. Similarly, in social interaction we need feedback from others so that we can judge how we are being received. This social feedback takes the form of verbal and nonverbal responses from those with whom we interact.

During interpersonal interaction a constant stream of feedback impinges upon the individual, both from the stimuli received from other people and from the physical environment. Not all of this feedback will be consciously perceived by the individual, since there is simply too much information to cope with. Thus a 'selective perception filter' (see Figure 4.6) is operative, and its main function is to filter a limited amount of information into the consciousness, while storing the remainder at a subconscious level. Evidence that such subconscious storage occurs can be seen during hypnosis, when the individual can recall information that he is not consciously aware of. The extent to which such subconscious information influences our behaviour is not clear, although judgements such as 'there was something about him I didn't like' may well be based upon subconscious perceptions.

As Figure 4.6 illustrates, from the large number of stimuli existing in the environment, a certain amount will be available as feedback to the individual, which will then be filtered into the consciousness or the subconscious. Within the physical environment the ticking of clocks, the hum of central heating systems, the pressure of one's body on the chair etc. are usually filtered into the subconscious during social encounters. However, if we are bored during an encounter e.g. sitting through a boring lecture, then these

Figure 4.6: Selective Perception Process

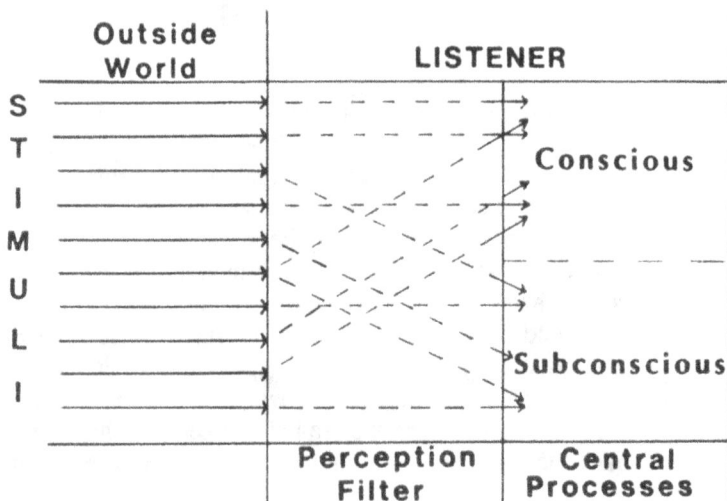

items may be consciously perceived and the social responses filtered into the subconscious. Unfortunately, during social interaction, vital information from another person may be filtered out and less important cues consciously perceived. In other words, from all of the feedback available to us, we may select less relevant stimuli to consciously perceive and miss the more important information. During SST, patients should learn to search for relevant interpersonal feedback, thereby ensuring that decisions about future responses are based upon valid incoming information.

Perception

Our perceptions, therefore, provide us with knowledge concerning the outside world. This knowledge is accumulated via the five sensory channels; sight, sound, touch, smell and taste. We use these channels to gather information both about physical objects and events, and about other people. As Warr and Knapper (1968) point out, 'person perception not only involves the judgements we make about people as objects (tall, bald, wearing brown shoes etc.) but is primarily concerned with the impressions we form of people as people (impulsive, religious, tired, happy, anxious and so on).' The importance of this dimension has been underlined by Cook (1979) who categorically states that, 'The way people see each other determines the way they behave towards each other, so the study of "person perception" is one of the keys to understanding social behaviour.' Thus, an awareness of some of the factors that influence the way in which we perceive others is of vital import in the study of social interaction.

Perceiving People and Objects

When we visit the cinema to watch a film, what we are actually 'seeing' is a series of still photographs shown in rapid sequence, which we then perceive as fluent motion. A similar phenomenon occurs with neon signs, where a series of bulbs lit in quick succession appears to us as the flowing movement of light. These are two simple examples of how we can be deceived by physical objects and events. Another example of how perception can be distorted is shown in the impossible figure in Figure 4.7. At first sight, this seems either like an object comprising three parallel tubes, or a magnet-like object, depending which end is focused upon. However, once the figure is perceived in its entirety it is realised that it is, in fact, an optical illusion rather than a repre-

Figure 4.7: Impossible Figure

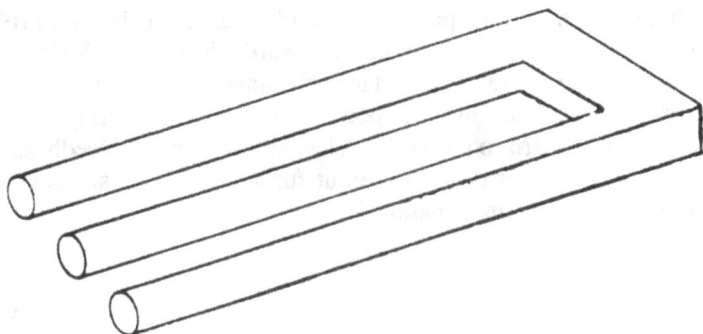

sentation of a real object. In person perception we can also be deceived by appearances. Family and friends may be shattered by someone who has committed suicide, since he or she may have seemed quite happy. Similarly, our initial perceptions of people we meet for the first time may later turn out to be quite inaccurate. Yet, as Arvey and Campion (1984) point out, important decisions such as whether or not to give someone a job, are often based on this type of first-impression judgement at selection interviews.

Our previous experiences also influence how we perceive the world, since we tend to select our perceptions to suit our expectations. This was illustrated in a study by Leeper (1935) who found that when shown the drawings in Figure 4.8, subjects were more likely to see an old woman in the ambiguous drawing (a) if they were shown (b) first, but were more likely to see a young woman in (a) if they were shown (c) first. Thus, we tend to search for perceptual cues which fit within our existing frame of reference. A similar process occurs in person perception, in that we can be 'taken in' by other people because we have certain pre-conceived views about them which influence how we actually perceive their behaviour. The wife who trusts her husband implicitly may not 'see' obvious signs that he is being unfaithful.

Roth (1976) has identified four important aspects of perception:

(1) Our perceptions enable us to structure and organise the world. Thus we respond to people as people, and not as a series of different shapes and colours

Figure 4.8: Old Woman/Young Woman

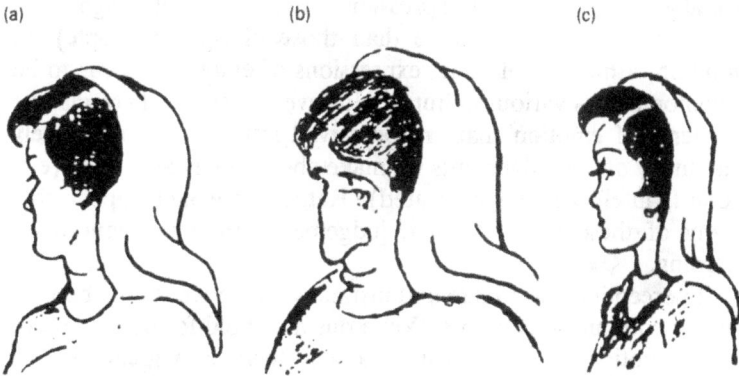

(a)   (b)   (c)

(2) We integrate a number of perceptual cues in order to make judgements. When we meet people we notice their dress, body shape, age, sex, voice and so on, and integrate all of this information to form an overall judgement

(3) We make associations and causal links between perceptions. Thus if we see a brick being thrown at a window we expect the glass to break, and interpret the breakage as being caused by the brick. Similarly, if we shout at someone and they cry, we assume our behaviour has caused them to cry

(4) We attribute stability and constancy to our perceptions. As people walk away from us they actually appear to get smaller, but we interpret this as being due to their distance from us and perceive them as still being the same height. We also look for stability and constancy in other people in that we expect people to adopt similar patterns of behaviour each time they meet us. In fact, we are surprised if this stability and constancy is missing in social encounters, as when a close friend is unexpectedly curt with us.

Theories of Perception

As Cook (1979) has illustrated, theories of perception can be divided into two main types, namely those that emphasise intuition, and those that emphasise inference. Intuitive theories regard perception as being innate, arguing that we instinctively recognise and interpret the behaviour and feelings of others. There is some evidence to support this viewpoint, in that monkeys reared in isolation are able to recognise and respond to the emotions being displayed by other monkeys. Also, humans blind from birth are able to display facial expressions of emotions (although these are more restricted in range than those of sighted people). In addition, a number of facial expressions of emotion appear to be common across various cultures. However, although there may be elements of emotion that are perceived intuitively, it is unlikely that many of the judgements we make about others are innate (e.g. honest, intelligent, sophisticated). Rather, it would appear that many of these more detailed judgements are dependent upon learning.

If perception was innate and instinctive, then we should be very accurate in our perceptions. While this may hold for perception of basic emotional states, such as anger, there is a great deal of research evidence to suggest that we are often very inaccurate in our perceptions. Furthermore, it has been demonstrated that it is possible to improve this accuracy of perceptions, thereby indicating that there is an element of learning involved in how we perceive the world. Thus, while it would appear that intuition has a role to play in perception, it is not sufficient to account fully for the overall process of perception.

The second theory purports that judgements about others are based on inferences made as a result of a number of perceptions, and that these are influenced by past experiences. An example of how this procedure would apply is as follows:

> Fat people are usually happy (generalisation based upon past experience)
> This woman is fat (this person is perceived as fitting the generalisation)
> Therefore she is probably happy (the inference is made).

It is clear that inferences will be stronger in some cases than in others. In particular, where inferences are based on objective criteria rather than on opinions, the inference can be made with more confidence. For example:

> All pupils at Newtown School wear a particular uniform
> He is wearing that uniform
> Therefore he is a pupil at Newtown School.

People seem to have 'implicit personality theories' (Bruner and Tagiuri, 1954) which they employ to make judgements about others. These theories seem to be dependent on three types of inference rules:

(1) Identification rules. These involve observing overt cues in order to identify people in certain ways (e.g. He is wearing a kilt, carrying a copy of the Scotsman, and speaking with a Scottish accent, therefore he must be Scottish!)
(2) Association rules. Once someone has been identified and placed in a certain category, they are associated with a set of other beliefs or stereotypes about the categorisation (e.g. He is Scottish, therefore he is probably careful with money)
(3) Combination rules. Perceptual cues need to be combined in order to make judgements. Where there are conflicting cues, judgements will be more difficult (e.g. He is wearing a kilt but speaking with a posh English accent. Is he Scottish upper-class, or English upper-class?).

It would therefore appear that both intuition and inference are important in person perception. The perception of certain basic emotions is probably important for the survival of the individual, but in a complex society, learned inferences will enable us to interpret a wide variety of social messages, and respond to these more readily. This means that it is possible to improve the perceptual ability of patients during SST.

Metaperception

As mentioned earlier, there are three main types of perception. In addition to the perception of other people, there is perception of self and metaperception. As we interact with others, we hear what we say to them and may be aware of some of our nonverbal responses. The socially skilled person will tend to be more aware of his own behaviour during social interaction, and will monitor and regulate his performance constantly in relation to the responses of others. However, it would seem that a curvilinear relationship exists between self-perception and social performance. Being excessively aware of oneself can be just as bad as being unaware of one's behaviour. People who are very self-conscious will not only display stilted social behaviour, they will also miss important cues from others.

Metaperception is the third aspect, and this refers to the perception of the perception process itself. When we interact with others we attempt to ascertain how they are perceiving us, and we try to evaluate how they think we are perceiving them. Both of these facets play an important role in interpersonal interaction. It has been shown that if person *A* likes *B* he will judge that *B* likes him. Furthermore, if *A* thinks *B* dislikes him he will tend to behave as if *B* did not like him, with the result that *B* will therefore probably not like him, and in this way a self-fulfilling prophecy occurs. There is evidence to suggest that perceptual inaccuracy is a feature of many patients. Neurotics tend to be more sensitive to cues of rejection but less sensitive to other perceptual cues. In schizophrenia, the selective perception filter can malfunction so that the person is flooded by stimuli from the outside world, and attempts to rectify this by 'switching off' and attempting to withdraw. Other general perceptual deficiencies amongst patients include paying attention to irrelevant cues, missing important cues, being easily distracted, having a short attention span, and selectively searching for cues that fit their view of the world.

Developing the ability of patients to perceive the cues being emitted by others more accurately, while being aware of their own responses, are both important dimensions of SST. To be effective in social interaction it is necessary to be sensitive to relevant social feedback, in terms of the verbal and nonverbal behaviour being displayed both by oneself and by others. If these perceptions are inaccurate, then decisions about future responses will be based upon invalid information, and the resulting responses are therefore likely to be inappropriate.

Situational Factors

In order to comprehend fully the behaviour of people during interpersonal encounters, it is necessary to consider the influence of situational factors. Magnusson (1981) argues that this is essential for three main reasons: we learn about the world and form conceptions of it in terms of the situations that we experience: all behaviour occurs within a given situation, and so cannot be fully understood without a knowledge of situational variables; by increasing our knowledge of situations we can increase our understanding of the behaviour of individuals.

Argyle et al (1981) define a social situation as 'the sum of the features of a social occasion that impinge on an individual'. They have identified nine main features of social situations:

Goal Structure

As discussed earlier, skilled behaviour is guided by goals, and no understanding of situations can be complete without a consideration of the goals being pursued by interactors. The goals being sought will be influenced by the situation in which one operates, and, also, we will seek out certain situations in order to attain certain goals. Thus, if we suddenly find ourselves being confronted by a very aggressive individual our immediate goal may be to ensure our personal safety. On the other hand, if it is our goal to find a mate we will seek out situations where we are likely to encounter members of the opposite sex.

Rules

Social interaction is often likened to a game in that both involve a set of rules that must be followed. The main difference is that games involve explicit rules, whereas most social rules are implicit. Nevertheless, it is important for people to adhere to the rules in any given social situation. Thus, it is not acceptable to listen to pop music on a radio in church, to refuse to answer any questions in a selection interview, or to serve yourself in a public bar. As Argyle et al (1981) have pointed out, it is often necessary to explain the rules of situations to patients in SST before teaching them the skills involved, just as one would explain the rules of squash to a novice before teaching him how to play certain shots.

Roles

In any given situation different individuals will play, and be expected to play, different roles. These roles carry with them a set of expectations about behaviour, attitudes, feelings and values. For example, a nurse is expected to behave in a thorough, professional manner, to care about patients' wellbeing, and attempt to help them overcome their problems. We play different roles from one situation to another, from nurse in the hospital to father in the home. We may also play more than one role in the same situation, so that if we have friends visiting we may play the roles of host, husband, and father. Patients should be aware of the range of roles, and their associated duties, which they and others may be expected to play in various situations.

Repertoire of Elements

Different types of behaviour will be more or less appropriate in different situations, and it is important for patients to learn which behaviours are relevant. The repertoire of elements suitable in any situation will also be dependent upon the specific goals of the individual. This is obviously a crucial aspect of SST programmes, and, in fact, forms the central component of such training. Chapters 7, 8 and 9 provide details of a range of behavioural elements.

Sequences of Behaviour

The elements of behaviour relevant to social situations usually occur in an expected sequence. At a simple level, one does not say 'goodbye' during greetings, or 'hello' during partings! Rather, behaviours are often performed in a pre-set, sequential, fashion. In certain instances, such as rituals or ceremonies, this can be a completely rigid and fixed sequence, as at a wedding in church. In other settings the sequence may be less formal, but still important. Going for a meal to a restaurant will usually involve:

(1) Entering the restaurant
(2) Going, or being shown, to a table
(3) Asking for, or being presented with, a menu
(4) Ordering the meal
(5) Being served
(6) Eating the meal
(7) Paying the bill
(8) Leaving the restaurant.

In addition, there are other elements that may be involved depending upon the way the situation unfolds (e.g. complaining about service or the meal).

Situational Concepts

A certain amount of conceptual information will be necessary for effective participation in each situation. In order to play soccer one must be aware of the concepts of 'off-side', 'throw in' and 'corner kick'. Similarly, in a restaurant one may need to be familiar with concepts such as 'hors d'ouvre', 'a la carte' and 'aperitif'.

Interestingly, different groups often use differing terms to describe the same concept (e.g. 'freedom fighters' as opposed to 'terrorists') so group members need to be aware both of appropriate concepts and their descriptors.

Physical Environment

The nature of an environment can have an influence upon the behaviour of the individual. People feel more comfortable and will tend to disclose more about themselves in warm environments (soft seats, concealed lighting, carpets, curtains etc.). Many patients will be unhappy having to interact in crowded environments, which have been shown to produce higher arousal, emotional discomfort, physical aggression and social withdrawal. How one manipulates interpersonal space will also influence social interaction, in that proximity can either be discomforting (too close or too distant) or facilitative (see Chapter 7).

Skills and Difficulties

Certain situations cause specific difficulties for individuals and therefore require special skills. For many people, selection interviews are very difficult and training will therefore be desirable. Patients will find certain situations more difficult than others, depending upon their level of skill in a particular context and their previous experience therein. The identification of problem situations for patients is therefore an important aspect of SST, since these situations will form an important component of study during training. Patients should learn skills appropriate to various situations and receive role-play practice in handling these situations. (Indeed, where possible the trainer should accompany the patient into various real situations at the final stage of training).

Language and Speech

There are linguistic variations associated with social situations; some situations require a higher degree of formality of language than others. Giving a lecture, being interviewed on television or chairing a committee meeting will all usually involve more formal, elaborate use of language as opposed to, for example, having a chat with a friend over coffee. Equally, changes in tone, pitch and volume of voice will change across situations. Thus, there are vocal patterns associated with clergymen giving sermons, barristers summing up, or commentators describing football games. Patients should recognise the importance of adjusting, as far as possible, their content and pattern of speech to meet the situation in which they operate.

These nine aspects of situations play an important role in interpreting the behaviour of individuals during social interaction. They should therefore be borne in mind during SST. Patients may have difficulties in social situations because of a misunderstanding of one or more of these aspects (such as breaking the rules, or not behaving in the expected sequence). Furnham (1983) reports the most commonly difficult situations for patients as being those involving intimacy, assertiveness, failure and rejection, being the focus of attention, complex social routines, pain and interpersonal loss. Elements of these situations will, for this reason, be a central focus during SST.

Personal Factors

The final element of the model of interpersonal interaction as outlined in Figure 4.3 relates to the personal factors of both individuals. By this we mean those aspects of each individual that are immediately visible to the other. Such factors include:

Sex

As Mayo and Henley (1981) point out, 'Sex as signaled by cues of appearance is a powerful force in human interaction ... and often the first aspect of another to which we respond'. We expect people to behave in certain ways depending upon whether they are male or female. Males are more likely to be viewed positively if they are seen as being competent, assertive and rational, whereas females are regarded positively if they display traits such as gentleness, warmth and tact. Clear differences can also be observed in the nonverbal behaviour of males and females, with the latter smiling more, requiring less interpersonal space, being touched more, using a greater number of head nods and engaging in more eye contact. Furthermore, women are also more skilled than men in interpreting nonverbal signals from others. The extent to which these differences are innate or learned remains unclear, although both of these dimensions are important in shaping gender differences in behaviour (Haviland and Malatesta, 1981). However, where males or females deviate markedly from the expected patterns of behaviour associated with their sex role, problems may arise in social interaction.

Physical Appearance

People are judged upon their appearance from a very early age. Nursery school children have been found to exhibit an aversion to chubby individuals, and a liking for physically attractive peers (Stewart et al, 1979). Teachers have also been found to attribute higher educational potential to attractive children. Attractiveness is therefore an important feature in social interaction. Cook (1977) in reviewing a number of facets of interpersonal attraction points out that:

> In most but not all relationships people look for someone who is attracted to them ... A relatively unattractive or unpopular person who tries to make friends with — or a sexual partner of — someone much more attractive or popular is likely to suffer a rebuff.

Someone regarded as being very attractive will also be seen as being popular, friendly, and interesting to talk to. This, in turn, will influence the way in which the attractive individual is approached by another person, thereby probably creating a self-fulfilling prophecy. Ratings of physical attractiveness seem to be consistent across variations in age, sex, socioeconomic status and geographical location, so that most of us will agree about the attractiveness of particular individuals. Marriage partners tend to be selected with this attractiveness criteria in mind, in that we will marry people at the same level of attractiveness as ourselves. Attractiveness, however, involves more than physical features, since other aspects such as cleanliness, dress, personality and competence are used in judging it. The latter two aspects will not be so important during initial encounters, but will be relevant in terms of the establishment of longer relationships.

Height and overall body shape will also have a bearing upon the behaviour of individuals. Height is certainly a significant element in judgements of males. Taller men tend to achieve more in our society in terms of occupational facets such as job opportunities, promotion and salary, and social facets such as dating. Higher status males are also viewed as being taller in direct proportion to their status, so that males of higher status are perceived as being taller. With females, it would seem that being tall is often regarded as a deficit, since 'short men and tall women have problems in date or mate selection ... when adolescent boys are worried about their height, they are worried by their shortness, whereas adolescent girls who worry about height are concerned by their tallness' (Stewart et al, 1979).

Physique can also influence how others are perceived and reacted to. For females, ectomorphs (thin figure) are rated most favourably, being seen as clean, tidy, quiet and conscientious, although nervous. Mesomorphic (muscular) females tend to be viewed as strong and healthy with a forceful personality, while endomorphs (fat) are often perceived as untidy, sloppy and lazy, although happy. With males, mesomorphs are most popular, followed by ectomorphs and, once again, endomorphs are least popular. Studies that have reported these findings have tended to concentrate on extreme stereotypes of body shape, and do not really consider variations within each stereotype. For example, a female with large breasts but a slim waist would not necessarily provoke the stereotype of an endomorph. Thus, more specific research is needed in this area before any firm conclusions can be reached with regard to reactions to specific body shapes.

Dress

Although one of the main functions of clothing is to protect the wearer from cold or injury, it is obvious that dress also serves a social function. The clothes we wear can serve to indicate group membership, individual identity, occupation, status, sex and personality. The amount of money spent annually in our society on clothes is a good indicator of the importance we attach to this aspect of appearance. In addition, we also employ other embellishments such as jewellery, expensive watches or carefully chosen spectacles to enhance our overall image. Since so much attention is devoted to the choice of dress, it is hardly surprisingly that we make judgements about others based upon this feature. Thus, Eicher and Kelley (1972) in a study of high school girls found that 'it is dress first, then personality, then common interests that lead to the pursual of friendships'. People who are well dressed and groomed are regarded as more socially competent.

Age

Although we may try to camouflage our actual age, for the most part this is something that can be accurately assessed by others, and is another feature of the person that will influence judgements. More mature professionals are often seen as being more competent, and so the newly qualified nurse may find difficulty in inspiring confidence in patients. Generally, we hold expectations about the behaviour of others based upon their age, and so we may regard an older person wearing trendy fashions as an 'old fool'. Indeed, 'act your age' is a maxim used to guide the behaviour of even young children! The problem age would appear to be late adolescence and early adulthood, when the individual is still developing a self-image, trying to establish a career and position in society, searching for a partner, or coping with the demands of a family. It is during this stage that problems such as schizophrenia, alcoholism or anorexia nervosa are most prevalent. Despite the often publicised problems of the elderly, 'The greatest life satisfaction is experienced by individuals who are approximately seventy years old. Although satisfaction declines after the age of seventy, it never reaches the low experienced by people in their twenties and thirties.' (Gergen and Gergen, 1981.)

These four features associated with the appearance of individuals need to be taken into consideration in any attempt to evaluate the process of interpersonal communication. The physical appearance and dress of patients are aspects that can be improved during SST. Encouraging patients to dress appropriately, use make-up to best advantage, or adopt a certain hair style are all legitimate strategies during SST. Improvements in overall appearance can result in increased perceptions of attractiveness which will, in turn, be very beneficial for patients during social encounters.

Overview

The model described in this chapter attempts to account for the central facets of interpersonal interaction. It will be apparent from the brief review of each of these facets that interaction between people is a complex process involving a myriad of variables, some, or all, of which may be operative at any particular time. Although each of these have been isolated for the purpose of analysis, it should also be realised that in reality these processes occur simultaneously. Furthermore, we are not usually aware that these processes are actually occurring, since we behave, for the most part, at a subconscious level. It is therefore extremely difficult to make judgements or interpretations about the exact reasons why certain behaviours are, or are not, displayed by individuals during social interaction. However, the model we have presented provides a systematic structure for interpreting human behaviour. This has incorporated an analysis of goals and motivation, cognition and emotion, social responses, feedback and perception, social situation, and personal factors, and of how these elements inter-relate.

Breakdown at any of the stages in this model will lead to impaired social performance, so patients should be made aware of the importance of each stage of the model. SST should therefore attempt either explicitly or implicitly, to effect patient competence at each stage. Thus, while social responses may be overtly addressed during SST, changes in patient cognitions may be indirectly effected by, for example, the use of questions by the nurse ('What might you have done?' 'What could you have changed?'). It is useful for patients to be given some form of theoretical underpinning for SST, and we would suggest that the model outlined in this chapter should be presented in an appropriate fashion to patients early in SST. This should help to place SST within a wider perspective, and thereby facilitate skill learning by patients.

5 DESIGNING AN SST PROGRAMME

In this chapter, the central elements involved in the design of an SST programme are presented. These are the features that need to be considered at the outset when preparing to employ SST in remediation, and they link closely with the factors discussed in Chapter 6 in relation to the actual operation of SST with psychiatric patients. In a sense, therefore, these two chapters should be taken together; they are separated mainly by the level of analysis. This chapter examines issues that would apply to SST in any number of settings in that it discusses the areas of assessment, training methods and techniques for facilitating transfer of learning. These issues are discussed particularly in the context of psychiatric nursing, but these are more fully explored in the following chapter. It is the intention of this chapter, therefore, to provide the reader with an understanding of the essential components of SST, as a pre-requisite to designing and implementing such a programme.

Assessment

Assessment in SST may be regarded as an extension of the initial overall assessment of the patient. Having identified that there may be certain social skill deficits, it is necessary to carry out a more systematic assessment in order to determine the exact nature and extent of a patient's problems. Such information is then used to make decisions about the content, methods and procedures to be employed in SST. At the assessment stage it is also possible to introduce patients to the concept of SST, and monitor their reactions to this form of training. There are eight main objectives of assessment, namely:

(1) To ascertain whether the patient is in need of SST
(2) To identify the specific social skill areas in which the patient is in need of improvement (as well as areas in which the patient has strengths)
(3) To decide whether or not an SST programme would be the

most appropriate method of remediation
(4) To provide the patient with information about the aims and procedures of SST
(5) To evaluate the patient's attitudes towards SST
(6) To ascertain whether the patient is willing to undertake a programme of SST
(7) To design an appropriate SST programme
(8) To collect baseline information about the patient, which can be compared against information gathered following SST.

If these assessment objectives are adhered to, and achieved, the SST programme will be built upon a solid foundation. While it is possible to organise and run SST programmes based on a general approach to understanding social interaction, the benefits of such an approach may well be minimal for patients. Such a generic approach may never really get to grips with the central problems encountered by the patient. Indeed, the adoption of a generic approach in SST may not only be detrimental to the patient, it may also serve to disillusion nursing personnel about the effectiveness and value of such a mode of treatment. (The application of such a 'watered-down' approach in the past may well have partially accounted for the lack of enthusiasm and support for innovations such as the therapeutic community and, more recently, the nursing process.) Furthermore, if a general approach to SST is employed, the nurse will not really have an in-depth understanding of the individual patient, which can only be obtained by detailed initial assessment. Another advantage of assessment is that attempting to understand fully the patient should inevitably help to develop the relationship between nurse and patient, thereby facilitating the interaction between the two. This can be a very important factor during the operation of SST when the nurse may have to provide negative, as well as positive, feedback to the patient.

Assessment Methods

There are a variety of assessment methods available for use in SST including staff questionnaires, self-report measures, interviews with patients and their peers or relatives, and observation of trainees. It is useful to examine each of these in more detail.

Staff Questionnaires.   This is a useful source of information about how the patient is viewed by those in authority, which in turn provides valuable information about how well, or poorly, the patient may interact with authority figures. Questionnaires can be given to staff who have spent some time interacting with or observing the patient, and will usually incorporate questions relating to both the behaviour and the attitudes of the patient. The design of questionnaires can probably best be undertaken using a multidiscipline approach, thereby drawing on expertise from a number of areas. A large number of different types of questionnaire can be used; one example is given in Figure 5.1, and further examples can be obtained from the references given at the end of this book. In designing a questionnaire to meet the needs of a specific situation, it should be kept simple, yet robust. In other words, it should not be offputting to those members of staff who will give their time to complete it, but at the same time it should provide enough information about the patient to be of value in making an assessment. Data obtained by this method are obviously subjective, each questionnaire representing the opinions of one particular person, and to glean as broad a perspective as possible it is useful to ascertain the views of various members of staff about any particular patient.

Self-report Measures.   Two main types of self-report measure can be employed, namely, questionnaires and sentence completion exercises. The object of both of these is to provide the patient with an opportunity of relating information about his or her thoughts, feelings and problems. They help the nurse to see, and attempt to make sense of, the world as viewed by the patient. Depending upon the context, one or other of these may be more applicable, but both are of value in building up a picture of the patient from his or her own perspective.

Questionnaires.   Again, this is a straightforward method of information gathering. As with all questionnaires various formats can be applied, for example the rating scale (see Figure 5.2). Here patients are asked to rate themselves on a number of factors, along a 3, 5, 6 or even 9 point Likert-type scale, where alternatives can range from, for example 'very strongly agree' to 'very strongly disagree' with a neutral mid-way point. An alternative format is to use the semantic differential method wherein the patient is asked to rate himself along a series of scales with opposing adjectives at either end, as in Figure 5.3. A third method is to use some form of

Figure 5.1: Staff Questionnaire

Patient_____ **Staff Member**_____ **Date**_____

On the basis of your knowledge of this patient please place a tick (✔) in the appropriate box opposite each of the following statements:

Relationships	Always	Often	Sometimes	Rarely	Never
1. Makes friends easily					
2. Is popular with other patients					
3. Is ignored by other patients					
4. Is aggressive with other patients					
5. Is easily influenced by other patients					
6. Has difficulty meeting strangers					
7. Readily joins in group activities					
8. Will initiate group activities					
9. Is friendly towards staff					
10. Is aggressive towards staff					
11. Accepts staff criticism					
12. Is willing to help staff					
13. Interacts easily with staff					
14. Will refuse staff instructions/requests					
15. Becomes annoyed if staff prevent him/her from doing something					
16. Seeks attention from staff					

Figure 5.2: Self Report Measures — The Likert-type Scale

Indicate your degree of agreement or disagreement with each of the following statements by circling one of the alternatives.

VSA — Very Strongly Agree
SA — Strongly Agree
A — Agree
U — Undecided
D — Disagree
SD — Strongly Disagree
VSD — Very Strongly Disagree

1.	I make friends easily	VSA	SA	A	U	D	SD	VSD
2.	I lose my temper quickly	VSA	SA	A	U	D	SD	VSD
3.	I find it difficult to talk to members of the opposite sex	VSA	SA	A	U	D	SD	VSD
4.	I enjoy going out shopping	VSA	SA	A	U	D	SD	VSD
5.	With strangers I often cannot think of anything to say	VSA	SA	A	U	D	SD	VSD
6.	I rarely feel embarrassed	VSA	SA	A	U	D	SD	VSD
7.	Other people do not really understand me	VSA	SA	A	U	D	SD	VSD
8.	I like going to parties	VSA	SA	A	U	D	SD	VSD
9.	I never feel depressed	VSA	SA	A	U	D	SD	VSD
10.	I am not very confident when talking to people	VSA	SA	A	U	D	SD	VSD
11.	I give in too easily to other people	VSA	SA	A	U	D	SD	VSD
12.	Other people seem to enjoy talking to me	VSA	SA	A	U	D	SD	VSD
13.	I do not enjoy speaking to a group of people	VSA	SA	A	U	D	SD	VSD
14.	I do not worry very much about anything	VSA	SA	A	U	D	SD	VSD
15.	I would describe myself as an attractive person	VSA	SA	A	U	D	SD	VSD
16.	I often make jokes and laugh with others	VSA	SA	A	U	D	SD	VSD
17.	I don't mind being criticised	VSA	SA	A	U	D	SD	VSD
18.	I often feel lonely	VSA	SA	A	U	D	SD	VSD
19.	I find it difficult to look directly at other people	VSA	SA	A	U	D	SD	VSD

Figure 5.3: Self-report Measures — The Semantic Differential

In each of the following place a tick (✔) at the point that best represents your point of view.

I see myself as being:

Worried	:____:____:____:____:____:____:____:	Carefree
Friendly	:____:____:____:____:____:____:____:	Unfriendly
Happy	:____:____:____:____:____:____:____:	Sad
Quiet	:____:____:____:____:____:____:____:	Talkative
Rude	:____:____:____:____:____:____:____:	Polite
Submissive	:____:____:____:____:____:____:____:	Assertive
Optimistic	:____:____:____:____:____:____:____:	Pessimistic
Attractive	:____:____:____:____:____:____:____:	Ugly
Nervous	:____:____:____:____:____:____:____:	Confident
Shy	:____:____:____:____:____:____:____:	Outgoing
Peaceful	:____:____:____:____:____:____:____:	Aggressive
Kind	:____:____:____:____:____:____:____:	Cruel
Tolerant	:____:____:____:____:____:____:____:	Intolerant
Fun-loving	:____:____:____:____:____:____:____:	Serious
Changeable	:____:____:____:____:____:____:____:	Always the same
Lazy	:____:____:____:____:____:____:____:	Industrious
Warm	:____:____:____:____:____:____:____:	Cold
Socially skilled	:____:____:____:____:____:____:____:	Socially unskilled
Boring	:____:____:____:____:____:____:____:	Interesting
Tense	:____:____:____:____:____:____:____:	Relaxed

check-list (see Figure 5.4) where the patient is presented with a list of problems and, for each, has to say whether or not it is a problem.

The type of questionnaire employed will depend upon the patient and the situation. Indeed, more than one type of questionnaire may be employed, since this exercise is not usually either too time-consuming, or too exhausting for the patient. Obviously, the language employed in the questionnaire has to be suitable for the patient and, where problems of literacy are encountered, the questionnaire may be used orally. If used in conjunction with staff questionnaires, it is possible to adjust the items slightly to have them included in both staff and self-report measures. This offers a useful comparison between the perceptions and perspectives of the patient and those of the members of staff. The actual selection of items for use in questionnaires is something that is difficult to dictate and at present, given the lack of validated instruments for use in SST, is almost a matter of trial and error. As long as questionnaires are used to facilitate the assessment process, and are not employed for research purposes, then this is a perfectly reasonable approach — and one which would appear to have been adopted by most practitioners.

Sentence completion. An alternative to the closed questionnaire method of assessment, this method is a more open-ended method. It consists of providing the patient with a few opening words to a sentence which he or she then completes. For example:

'I am the type of person who ....'
'My main problems at the moment are ....'
'The things I would like to change about myself are ....'
'My main strengths are ....'

The list of openings is virtually limitless, and may be geared to specific situations or general areas, as above. The advantage of this approach is that it allows the patient complete freedom of expression. In practice, some patients will find difficulty with a completely open approach, and may need guidance when using this method. Where there are problems of literacy this can be presented orally and patient responses either written down or audio-recorded (with prior consent). Thus, with some patients it may be sufficient to give them a sheet of paper with the opening to a

Figure 5.4: Self-report Measures: A Problem Checklist

For each of the following statements place a tick (✔) to indicate whether this is never a problem, sometimes a problem or often a problem.

	Never a problem	Sometimes a problem	Often a problem
1. Meeting strangers			
2. Saying 'no' to other people			
3. Talking to members of the opposite sex			
4. Losing my temper			
5. Going shopping			
6. Going to parties			
7. Going to the pub			
8. Feeling depressed			
9. Feeling anxious			
10. Understanding what other people are thinking about			
11. Being humorous			
12. Thinking of things to say to other people			
13. Looking at other people			
14. Getting other people to understand me			
15. Feeling lonely			
16. Making friends			

17. Lacking confidence			
18. Going into a room full of people			
19. Accepting criticism			
20. Going for an interview			

sentence at the top and ask them to complete it, whereas with others it may be necessary to talk through it (by giving examples of 'types of problems' or 'strengths').

Interviews. This assessment technique does not really need detailed description, since it will be very familiar to psychiatric nurses. There are a few points that should be borne in mind however. Firstly, the interview should be structured in such a fashion as to elucidate the central problems encountered by the patient. Secondly, the nurse should be skilled at probing for depth of analysis, so that the patient, peers or relatives are encouraged to discuss the patient's problems fully. Finally, it is important that concrete information is obtained, rather than generalities. For example, if a patient reports that he or she 'gets anxious when meeting strangers', this should be explored further in order to ascertain what exactly the patient *does* in terms of meeting strangers.

Observation of Patients. The most direct method for assessing patients is to observe them interacting. However, there are a number of difficulties associated with this method. The first decision that has to be made is whether to observe the patient in 'real' or 'contrived' settings or in role-plays. Observation in real settings would take place by watching the patient interact with other patients, ward staff or relatives. This may encompass either real settings within the clinic or ward, for hospitalised patients, or real settings in the patient's own environment. While the latter may be more difficult to arrange, it may provide greater insight into the patient's problems. Contrived settings involve recruiting an accomplice (usually another member of staff) to interact with the patient, without the patient being aware that this has been contrived. In both the two settings, there is an ethical dilemma of whether or not to observe the patient 'surreptitiously'. If the patient is later told that such observation has taken place, it may affect the level of trust placed in the nurse.

It is possible, of course, to inform the patient in advance that observation will take place. The problem then is that a knowledge of being observed can distort the natural pattern of patient behaviour, and so invalidate the observations. In practice both of these methods are often difficult to carry out, and the role-play method is commonly used. This involves setting up a range of problem situations in which the patient interacts with people (other patients or staff) who play various roles (e.g. shop assistant, possible date, parent). One advantage of this approach is that, with the patient's agreement, the role-plays can be video-recorded for detailed analysis and evaluation. It also circumvents the ethical problem inherent in naturalistic observation. A major disadvantage is that the behaviour of patients in role-play may differ from that which they display in reality. There is some evidence to suggest that by providing detailed background descriptions and infor-mation to role-players, the validity of this technique can be improved. Nevertheless, it should be taken as an indicator, rather than an actual record, of patient behaviour.

A behavioural evaluation of the patient can also be made by participant observation. For example, when using the interview method of assessment it is possible to gather information regarding patient behaviour. The problem with participant observation is that it is difficult simultaneously to participate with and closely observe and analyse the patient. Nevertheless, general impressions can be obtained using this method (e.g. 'never smiles', 'avoids eye con-tact'), although a detailed assessment of behaviour cannot. One compromise here is to obtain the permission of the patient to video-record assessment interviews, thereby obtaining a record of interaction for later analysis. A further advantage is that this method provides baseline behavioural data with which to evaluate the effects of SST, as well as facilitating the goals of training.

A number of methods exist for the analysis of behavioural data. One is to use some form of rating system, whereby the patient is rated, usually by members of staff, on a 5 or 7 point scale on a number of behaviours, as in Figure 5.5. This provides a qualitative record of how the patient is viewed by independent observers. As with all qualitative analyses, such ratings are subjective, and for ratings to be valid and reliable, extensive training of observers is

Figure 5.5: A Rating System for Analysis of Patients' Nonverbal
Behaviours

For each of the following non-verbal features, place a circle around the number that
best represents your judgement of this patient:

	Never appropriate	Seldom appropriate	Erratic use of	Usually appropriate	Always appropriate
Dress	1	2	3	4	5
Eye contact	1	2	3	4	5
Posture	1	2	3	4	5
Hand movements	1	2	3	4	5
Smiles	1	2	3	4	5
Facial expressions (other than smiles)	1	2	3	4	5
Interpersonal distance	1	2	3	4	5
Touch	1	2	3	4	5
Physical appearance (hair, make-up, cleanliness)	1	2	3	4	5

required. However, for training purposes, ratings can be used as general indicators of how well, or poorly, the patient uses certain behaviours. An alternative to ratings is to use a system of frequency counts, where a behaviour is given a score of one every time it is used by the patient. Thus, for example, a score of the total number of questions, interruptions or self-disclosures can be made. Certain behaviours lend themselves more easily to this type of frequency analysis than others. For example, it can be very difficult to count eye contact, smiles and head nods. An alternative is to use a time-line display as in Figure 5.6. Here a sheet is divided up into a number of 15 or 30-second intervals and the behaviour is scored once if it occurs during any interval. While this record may be less exact than frequency counts for certain behaviours it is more easily scored, and it does provide a useful indicator of the extent to which a particular behaviour is employed.

Thus, the type of observation method used is dependent on both the behaviour to be observed, and the function of the observation. Indeed, various types of observation system may be employed in order to build up a picture of the behavioural style of the patient. For example, in relation to patient talk, a stop watch may be utilised to measure overall volume of talk, ratings can be

Figure 5.6: The Interval Method for Scoring Patient Nonverbal Behaviour

For each of the following behaviours score (✔) only once if the behaviour occurs during each 30-second interval, otherwise leave blank.

Time intervals	1	2	3	4	5	6	7	8	9	10	11	12
Head nod												
Smile												
Hand movement (communicative)												
Hand movement (self-directed)												
Movement of legs/feet												
Posture shift												
Eye contact												

obtained of vocal variation, and frequency counts made of self-disclosures, interruptions or questions. A number of observation systems have been developed to facilitate such analyses, including a fairly extensive range of assessment scales by Spence (1980).

Planning SST Programming

Following the detailed assessment of the patient, the next step is to plan an appropriate SST programme to meet the assessed needs. There are two main stages involved here. Firstly, setting and agreeing the training goals, and secondly, identifying appropriate training methods.

Setting Training Goals

Two of the objectives given earlier for assessment were to evaluate the patient's attitude to SST and to determine whether the patient is willing to undertake a programme of SST. These would usually be incorporated into the interview with the patient. During the interview, the basic rationale behind SST would be explained, and emphasis placed upon the necessity for willingness on the part of the patient to participate, as a pre-requisite to running the programme. Without such willingness, SST will not usually be undertaken by the nurse. Since this method of training can be very demanding for the patient (even for one who is keen to participate!), lack of initial commitment can lead to early withdrawal from the SST programme, and time and effort for everyone involved is wasted. While assessment of the patient is a normal part of the nursing process, the detailed behavioural assessment already outlined may not take place if the patient indicates a reluctance to enter into SST.

Once SST has been explained and the patient agrees to participate, the emphasis should be on as open an approach to training as possible. It is this openness that is one of the characteristic features of SST and sets it apart from other approaches to remediation (such as behaviour modification). The methods and functions of the assessment phase should be presented, and permission obtained to implement whichever methods are decided upon. In this sense a contract is being entered into between nurse and patient, and this can be either oral or written, depending upon the patient. The written contract should, as in Figure 5.7, cover both

Figure 5.7: SST Agreement Form

I agree to undertake a programme of social skills training organised by

_____.

I understand that this SST programme will involve a period of assessment and I hereby give permission to have my behaviour observed by the above trainer/s. I also give permission to have my behaviour video-taped during practicals. I understand that at no time will my behaviour be recorded on audio- or video-tape without my full prior knowledge. I also understand that all material recorded on tape will be treated as strictly confidential, and will not be shown to anyone outside the training situation without my written approval. I undertake to give my full commitment to the SST programme.

PATIENT:_____ DATE_____

       TRAINER/S_____

                _____

                _____

assessment and video-recording elements of SST as well as underline the patient's commitment to the programme. Obviously, an oral contract would also incorporate all of these elements and can be more appropriate if the intention is to develop a degree of informality into the training environment, while maintaining the patient's level of trust and confidence in the trainer.

The goals set for SST should be patient-orientated rather than programme-based, in that the programme should be adjusted to fit the requirements of the patient. Where a group, rather than individual, approach to training is being used, patients with similar problems should be grouped together for training. This also means that the goals will be dependent upon the type of patient (i.e. short or long-stay) and the situation in which they operate (community or ward). This issue will be explored more fully in Chapter 6.

The data accumulated during the assessment phase will then be used to set goals for the training programme. These goals may relate directly to specific behavioural difficulties experienced by the patient, for example:

(1) To improve the ability of Mr X to maintain appropriate eye contact during conversation
(2) To improve the ability of Ms A to speak in a normal tone of voice rather than in a whisper
(3) To enable Mr Y to be able to open an appropriate conversation with a stranger.

Goals may also be related to internal states, such as:

(4) To develop in Mr B a sense of critical awareness, both of himself and of others, in social interaction
(5) To increase the confidence of Mr C when participating in groups
(6) To help Ms D improve her level of self-esteem.

Behavioural goals are more amenable to direct measurement and evaluation, whereas goals related to internal states need to be measured indirectly. Thus, while it is possible to observe the level of eye contact of a patient, their level of confidence is measured by using either some form of questionnaire or interview procedure. Nevertheless, both sets of goals are important and should be included in any SST programme. Cognitions and emotions are directly linked with behaviour, and so a knowledge of all three elements is needed to gain a full understanding of the patient and how he has been influenced by SST. When a complete set of goals has been formulated, these should be fully agreed by the patient as appropriate before embarking upon SST practice.

Training Methods

Following the agreement about the goals of SST, the next step is to design a programme of training, tailored to achieve these goals. When designing such a programme there are a number of central elements that are crucial to the successful implementation of SST. The elements are, in effect, the defining characteristics of SST and include sensitisation, modelling, behaviour rehearsal, role-play, types of feedback, the use of closed circuit television (CCTV), homework and facilitating transfer.

Sensitisation

Sensitisation refers to the phase in SST when the patient is introduced to the aspects to be studied during each session. The first practical session of SST is of crucial importance, since this will set the scene for the remainder of the programme and provide the patient with an indication of what to expect in future sessions. For this reason, it is important to structure carefully the initial session in such a way as not to overload the patient in a new and unfamiliar training setting, yet cover enough to indicate that SST will be a worthwhile experience. In the first session, therefore, the following areas can be covered:

(1) The objectives of SST. Although these have already been agreed, it is useful to restate them at the outset. In group SST work, these can be put on a handout, overhead projector or flip chart, to facilitate group involvement.
(2) The rationale behind SST. Again, this should have been explained beforehand, and it is a matter here of underlining what SST can and cannot offer the patient. Any unrealistic patient expectations need to be identified at this juncture.
(3) Emphasis on patient involvement and commitment. It is important to emphasise that the patient will be expected to participate fully in SST, and that failure so to do will adversely effect any benefits to be gained from training. The nurse should also state their own degree of commitment and enthu-

siasm at this stage, and explain the nature of SST as a joint venture between patient and nurse.

(4) Outline of proposed programme. The nurse should provide, again using audio-visual aids, a basic outline of the SST programme, explaining timing and content. In addition, methods of teaching should be briefly explained, in terms of aspects such as use of role-play, behaviour rehearsal, feedback from nurse, peers or CCTV, and homework.

(5) Group familiarisation. When operating a group SST programme it is important to have an exercise wherein members begin to get to know one another (if they do not already do so). There are numerous methods whereby this can be achieved. One approach is to split the group into pairs. The individuals in each pair find out from one another certain basic information (name, home location, etc.), and the group then comes back together and person A introduces person B to the group, relating the gathered information; B then introduces A, and so on.

(6) CCTV familiarisation. If CCTV is to be utilised, then it is important to introduce patients to this medium as early as possible. Depending upon the time available, this can be achieved either in the first or the second session. CCTV is often the most anxiety-provoking feature of SST, so great care must be taken when employing this method of feedback. However, if patients have agreed to its use then it is important to provide early exposure for two reasons. Firstly, to prevent a build-up of worry regarding its impending usage on the part of patients, which may interfere with initial attention and learning. Secondly, to identify those patients who may suffer adversely from video-feedback and, if necessary, adjust the programme for such patients (if necessary, by eliminating CCTV). The first exposure to CCTV should be both relaxed, fairly brief, and not focused on the individual behaviour of any patient. This can be achieved by video-taping a segment of a group discussion with the camera encompassing all of the group for most of the time, but then zooming in on each patient for a short period (5 — 10 seconds). This is replayed to the group simply to let them see themselves. Patients can be encouraged to express their initial reactions to self-viewing, and these reactions should be carefully monitored. At this stage a 'cosmetic shock' usually occurs, with most people being

surprised by their appearance and voice, and this should be pointed out to patients. This video playback session should be kept totally relaxed, and no detailed analysis of patient behaviour should be entered into. Other aspects of CCTV will be further explored later in this chapter.

After the first session, the patient should be fully aware of what SST will involve, and familiar with the overall approach to training, the nurse, other patients involved and CCTV (time permitting). Each following session should begin with a recap of what has been learned in previous sessions, followed by a discussion of what is to be covered in the forthcoming session. This lets patients know where they have been, where they are now, and where they are going. This sensitisation stage should not be rushed through since it is important to lead patients into the social skill to be covered, so that they are fully prepared for what is to follow. For example, if the topic is eye contact, the nurse may introduce this by asking questions such as 'How do you feel if you are talking to someone and they never look at you?' 'Do you look more at people when you are speaking or when they are speaking?' 'What will happen if you continually stare at a complete stranger?' Questions such as these can be explored in depth as a prelude to a practical on the use of eye contact.

Modelling

Following the sensitisation of patients to the area under focus, the next step is to provide some form of model of the behaviour in action. Modelling is the process whereby the patient observes a demonstration of the behaviour as displayed by someone else. There are a variety of types of model that can be employed in SST, including the following.

Live Trainer Modelling. Here the trainer demonstrates to patients the behaviour being discussed. Thus, for example, the nurse may exemplify various types of posture and have patients discuss the meaning of each. This method has the advantage of being easy to organise, is often stimulating for patients, and can also indicate to the patient that the nurse is a skilful individual who can practise what he or she preaches. The main disadvantage is that the patient may give the 'it's easy for him' response, by not identifying with the nurse as someone in a similar situation or facing the same problems.

Live Peer Modelling.   Other patients can be used to model particular behaviours. The potency of this approach can be recognised by the fact that much of the institutional-type of behaviour encountered on long-stay wards is the result of live peer modelling, wherein patients acquire socially inappropriate behaviours by modelling other patients. During SST, the nurse needs to be certain that the patient chosen to be the model is capable of displaying the behaviours. This approach can be very rewarding for the 'model' patient, and has the advantage of providing a model with which the other patients can identify. One disadvantage is that it can make the patients who have difficulty with these behaviours feel inferior to the model, and can even provoke jealousy.

Taped Models.   The use of audio- or video-taped models is common practice in SST. The advantage of these as opposed to live models is that they can be carefully prepared and structured in advance. There are a number of commercially available audiovisual packages available, but in practice these are rarely completely appropriate for any given situation, and it is better to try to produce tailor-made model tapes. These do not need to be technically perfect, so long as the behaviours being exemplified can be clearly seen and heard. The production of video models only necessitates a camera, microphone (this may be built-in to the camera), video recorder and actors (usually other members of staff unknown to the patients in SST). Audio models obviously require only an audio-recorder and actors. Time spent in producing taped models is worthwhile since these facilitate an in-depth analysis of behaviour, in that critical elements can be played, discussed and reviewed. The teaching of nonverbal behaviours is greatly facilitated by video, where the action can be 'stilled' for evaluation of particular behaviours. Similarly, if the emphasis is on vocals (pitch, tone, volume, speed, etc.) then audio-tape is very useful and the video element not so essential.

Diagrammatic Models.   This includes the use of diagrams, illustrations and photographs. Such methods are especially useful when discussing aspects of nonverbal communication. Photographs of facial expressions are widely employed in SST, as are matchstick-men diagrams to demonstrate various postures, and illustrations of seating arrangements around a table. These are not only useful teaching aids, they also add variety, and stimulate the learning process.

Symbolic Models. This refers to all forms of written material designed to inculcate skill, knowledge and awareness. It would include summative handouts describing the skill, or the use of books for patients to read. Another type of symbolic model is to provide a written transcript of an interaction sequence, and have patients analyse this in terms of, for example, use of questions or self-disclosures.

Depending upon the ability of patients, resources available and training goals, a variety of these types of model can be used during training. A number of factors need to be considered when preparing models for use in SST:

(1) The model must be similar to the patient in terms of age, sex, race and socio-economic background. In other words, the patient must be able to identify readily with the model and this is where commercially produced video packages can often fail. The authors have discovered that in Northern Ireland, for example, to be effective models should ideally be seen as Northern Irish, although Scottish, Northern England and Southern Irish models are fairly acceptable. Models from Canada, USA, Australia or the South of England are not identified with to the same extent, and do not provide as valuable a learning experience.
(2) The model should be portrayed as facing similar problems to those faced by the patient. Again, this is important from the point of view of identification with the model.
(3) Most of the models used should demonstrate positive examples of the skill, although negative examples can also be employed. Research findings in this field are equivocal, with contradictory results relating to the influence of negative models. The argument most often employed against negative models is that the patient may learn to use inappropriate behaviour displayed by the model. On the other hand, it is argued that patients need to learn what is inappropriate as well as what is appropriate if they are to become more socially skilled. It would seem that a possible solution is to ensure that

the patient is fully aware of when models are being used inappropriately and is encouraged to discuss why they are inappropriate. Such models, therefore, must be *clearly* inappropriate. The emphasis, however, should be on providing a majority of positive models, and the models should be seen as being rewarded for displaying appropriate behaviours.

(4) Models should be seen as 'coping' rather than as perfect. The model should be portrayed as someone gradually overcoming their problems, rather than as someone with no problems in social interaction.

(5) Models should be as varied as possible. If the same person is constantly portrayed as the model, this can become tedious for patients and reduce the modelling potential. The use of various people as models can emphasise the fact that problems are shared by many, and can increase the learning of patients. By using a range of models, the likelihood is also increased that the patient will identify strongly with some of these, whereas if one model is used and the patient does not identify with it then the effort is largely wasted.

The modelling phase of training is crucially important, since it is at the sensitisation and modelling stages that skills are actually learnt, and often it is only when the patient sees the skill in action that such learning occurs. As much time as is deemed necessary should therefore be spent on the analysis and discussion of models. While taped models should be kept fairly brief (certainly no longer than 5 minutes), these can be paused or replayed for further discussion. One technique here is to use the 'What should happen next?' or 'What did you think of that?' type of question after stopping the tape at a critical point in the interaction. This encourages critical analysis, and helps to develop the cognitive capacity of patients for monitoring social situations.

Practice

When the skill under focus has been assimilated by patients, the next step is to allow them to practise it. Successful practice reinforces any skill learning that has taken place, and serves to increase the confidence of the patient. The distinction between skill learning at a conceptual level and ability to put the skill into practice should be clearly recognised. Thus, the patient may recognise the importance of eye contact and be able to verbalise important aspects concerning its usage, but may not be able to implement appropriate eye contact during social interaction practicals. In such instances, repeated practice and feedback should result in behavioural improvement. Two main types of practical can be employed in SST.

Behaviour Rehearsal. As the name suggests, this comprises simply having the patient practise (rehearse) the behaviour during training. Some behaviours lend themselves more to this direct form of practice. For example, eye contact, smiles, head nods, posture, giving verbal rewards and improving vocalisations (e.g. by reading a passage aloud) can be trained using behaviour rehearsal. Targets can be set for patients to achieve where objective measures can be obtained, such as: 5 seconds of continuous eye contact; one head nod every 10 seconds; or one verbal reward after receiving a response. Where targets are set it is important that the patient is capable of achieving them since failure can be counter-productive. Targeting is particularly useful where the behaviour is not being displayed by the patient, since it simply encourages the patient to try out the behaviour. Once the behaviour has been established then appropriate usage can be encouraged by other methods.

Role-play. The advantage of role-plays is that they take into account the appropriateness of behaviour as well as amount. In other words, they emphasise the quality as well as the quantity of responses. Situations to be role-played should resemble as closely as possible the situations in which patients will interact, and indeed can be based upon problems they have encountered. They should also have a gradation of difficulty, moving from simple situations early in training to more complex ones later. In addition, it is advisable to have closely structured role-plays in the early stages, involving detailed written or verbal descriptions of the roles to be played, together with extensive discussion with the participants about how the situation will develop, what responses each should make and how the role-play will come to an end (Milroy, 1982). Such an approach is useful if the patients have not been involved in role-plays before, and if this is the case it is likely that patients may find difficulty getting into their roles. The nurse should also be prepared to engage in role-plays, partly to avoid the 'me and them' syndrome in training, and partly to demonstrate how a role can be effectively portrayed. The nurse, however, should play a subsidiary role and as training progresses should withdraw from direct involvement in role-play. As a general rule, it is important not to expect too much too soon from this training technique.

As training progresses, patients become more experienced and role-plays can become less structured and may involve no more than a brief introductory description, for example:

Person A: You are standing in a supermarket check-out queue in somewhat of a hurry since you have a lot of groceries and are worried about missing your bus. You are just about to pass your groceries to the cashier.

Person B: You are in a supermarket ready to check-out with your groceries. You are in a hurry, since you had agreed to pick your husband up in the centre of town. It is raining and you are already late. You go to the shortest queue where there is only one person waiting. Open the conversation by walking in front of A and saying 'You don't mind me going in front of you, do you, but I'm in a desperate rush'.

In this situation, the assertive skills of A would be under focus.

Role-plays should allow patients to face both sides of a difficult situation, since this encourages them to see the other person's point of view. The ability to take the role of another person and see the world through their eyes is used as a test of social sensitivity and is, in itself, a valuable experience. Thus, patients may be required to ask for a date or be asked for a date, be interviewed for a job or act as a job interviewer. The nurse must be sensitive at all times during role-plays, and be prepared to cut the action if anyone is suffering, or if things are not going as planned. If necessary, the role can be broken down into smaller elements and each practised separately.

Following role-plays, there should be a period of 'de-roleing', when patients are permitted to come out of the role and be themselves again. During this stage the patient should be encouraged to relate his or her feelings immediately upon termination of the role, and gradually begin to discuss his or her performance more objectively by using terms such as 'in the role' or 'as interviewer'. Detailed feedback to role-players is essential in order to maximise learning. Feedback is facilitated by audio or video-recording, but this is not essential since feedback from other sources can be utilised. Where the patient has not been successful during a role-play, it may be useful to allow him or her to try again following feedback, especially if there is a good chance of successful practice second time round.

Feedback

As explained in Chapter 4, feedback is a crucial process in learning any new skill or technique. Without some form of feedback, learning will not usually take place. It is therefore important to pay close attention to the provision of feedback to patients during SST. For feedback to be effective, it should be given as soon as possible after the patient has been involved in practical exercises. This applies equally to video feedback which, in theory, could be delayed for a long period. The effects of such delays, however, would be to interfere with intervening patient activities and reduce the learning benefits. There are four main types of feedback for use during SST.

The Nurse. As trainer in SST, the nurse is a very potent source of feedback. He or she must have the ability not only to reward the patient for successful practice, but also sensitively to provide negative feedback when the patient has not successfully displayed the behaviours under analysis. Regardless of how poorly the patient may have performed, however, it is vital that he or she receives some positive feedback (e.g. for effort, motivation or willingness to participate). This positive feedback should always be provided before going on to discuss unsuccessful aspects of performance. When discussing these unsuccessful aspects the nurse should attempt to ascertain from the patient possible reasons for lack of success, before suggesting how the patient could improve. It is important to discover if the patient has recognised the lack of success, without having to be told, and if so it is useful to see whether the patient has any ideas about why they were not successful, and suggestions about how to improve. This is sometimes referred to as the 'Listen → Tell' approach to supervision, and is intended to improve the ability of patients to monitor their own performance.

Although the primary focus of attention should be upon behavioural components, the thoughts and feelings of patients should also be explored during feedback discussions since these play a central role in determining social responses (see Chapter 4). However, the main emphasis should be on the behaviours under review for that session. Reference can also be made to behaviours already covered during SST, in order to encourage an integrated approach to training. In addition, a more direct form of feedback can be given to the patient during practicals, whereby the nurse provides instant feedback to the patient during an interaction. In its basic form this can involve the nurse sitting or standing near the patient and whispering information to him or her. A less obtrusive method is to provide the patient with an ear-piece attached to a microphone through which the nurse can provide prompts from a distance (preferably from another room with one-way mirror or camera link). These methods are generally only recommended where the patient has extreme difficulty in learning a particular skill, and such prompting should be withdrawn as soon as possible, with the emphasis being placed upon patient independence and responsibility for their own behaviour.

Other Patients.   Feedback can be obtained from other patients during group SST sessions. One advantage here is that it encourages patients to observe and analyse social interaction, and this can be a valuable learning experience in itself. Patient feedback must be carefully supervised by the nurse, however, especially if it is becoming too negative. Patients can certainly be involved in providing quantitative feedback, for example by using a stopwatch to time the duration of talk or eye contact, counting number of questions, verbal rewards or self-disclosures. Such activities also serve to increase the involvement of patients when they are not directly participating in practicals.

Audiovisual.   Perhaps the most powerful form of feedback available is to use CCTV and video replays. The use of video in mental health practice is an issue that is receiving increasing attention (Heilveil, 1983) without any hard and fast conclusions yet being reached. There are a number of advantages and disadvantages associated with this medium. The advantages of using video during SST are:

(1) It is a valuable tool with which to gain the attention and maintain the motivation of patients. Especially during the initial stages of training, video will be a novel feature of training for many patients who will be highly motivated when performing 'on camera'.
(2) It provides both instant and accurate feedback. Once a role-

play has been completed it can be replayed immediately to let patients see how they have performed, and to see themselves as others see them. The fact that the camera does not lie is also useful in situations where the patient may deny using a particular behaviour. In such instances where video is used 'in evidence' against the patient, tact and sensitivity are obviously needed when confronting the patient with examples of the behaviour being denied. In this way, video can help overcome arguments between nurse and patient regarding what actually happened during practicals. It is also valuable in that it can help the patient to recognise what they are doing wrong, and this is a pre-requisite to accepting the need for change.

(3) Video playback facilitates an in-depth analysis of behaviour. Once a tape has been recorded it can be played and critical elements of it can be reviewed; it can be played in slow motion or the action frozen for closer analysis of nonverbal components. In this way, an extensive evaluation of the patient can be made, both qualitative and quantitative.

(4) The use of video encourages a sense of critical self-awareness on the part of the patient, which would otherwise be very difficult to achieve. Being able to see and hear oneself interacting is a memorable experience for most people. At the very least, patients will become aware of their own physical appearance. Most patients will eventually go beyond a concern with their physical image to begin to analyse and evaluate their own style of interacting.

The main disadvantages with video are:

(1) It is anxiety-provoking. Research findings have clearly shown that the use of video increases the anxiety levels of those exposed to this medium. For patients with existing high levels of anxiety, being video-taped may be a very frightening experience. Great care needs to be exercised when using video with such patients, and at all times participation in exercises involving video-taping should be voluntary.

(2) It can provide negative cosmetic feedback. With elderly patients, or patients with physical disfigurements, self-viewing on video can be a very negative experience. If there is a danger of patients suffering unduly because of their physical appearance, video should not be used during SST.

(3) Patients may find negative performance feedback difficult to accept. Indeed, there is evidence to suggest that some patients will operate cognitive defensive mechanisms during self-viewing, whereby they distort or interpret information received from video in such a fashion as to refuse to accept personal responsibility for their behaviour. The behaviour may be attributed to the presence of the camera itself or the artificiality of the situation. In such instances the nurse should acknowledge that the camera can influence behaviour, as can the artificiality of the training environment, and show understanding of the patient's feelings. Often, the patient can be encouraged to analyse their own behaviour in the context of such possible distortions, by talking through how they may affect them.

(4) Video-playback can result in a process known as 'self-confrontation'. This occurs when the ideal self-image of the patient is challenged by the public image as portrayed on the TV screen. Quite often a mis-match will occur between the self-image of an individual and the image presented on video. This can be very traumatic for patients, who may respond in a number of ways. Some patients will be determined to try to improve their performance so that the ideal and real images come closer together. Others will simply reject the public image as being a distortion. Finally, some patients may be adversely affected by, for example, increased withdrawal, bizarre behaviour or self-deprecation. Research in the clinical setting is inconclusive on what effects video-playback will have with various types of patient. Undoubtedly, an important factor here is the manner in which video is introduced, operated, and used as a feedback tool.

The nurse must be very sensitive to patient reactions at all times, and if a patient is becoming very uncomfortable, then the video replay should be terminated and alternative feedback given. As mentioned earlier, exposure to video should be gradual, with a very brief period being given initially. Patients should always be encouraged to talk through their reactions to video, and given help in overcoming any negative experiences. The confidentiality of video-tapes should be ensured, and, if necessary, the patient should be allowed to see tapes being erased.

Where video cannot be used, for whatever reason, it may be

possible to employ audio-recording as a source of feedback. Audio-feedback is much less anxiety-provoking, but obviously also contains must less information. It is useful for dealing with verbal skills such as asking questions, giving rewards, using reflections, self-disclosing, and explaining; or vocal skills such as tone, pitch, volume, speed, pauses and interruptions. One advantage here is that sometimes the nonverbal information available on video can be a distraction when analysing verbals and vocals, and audio-tape allows for more concentrated feedback. Conversely, a disadvantage is that often the verbal and vocal information under study can only be fully understood in the context of accompanying nonverbal information.

Observation Records. In order to provide focused feedback during SST, some form of observation schedule to facilitate analysis and evaluation is often useful. There is evidence to suggest that such a method improves the learning of social skills. Observation schedules can consist simply of a number of headings on a sheet of paper, listing the main behaviours under focus for one particular session. It is recommended that no more than four central behaviours be studied during any one session, and if the behaviour is complex or if the patient has particlar problems with it then it should be taken as a separate unit of analysis. Other forms of observation records can be made, including frequency counts or timing the duration of behaviour. The advantage of this type of quantitative data is that it provides a concrete record for comparison over time.

Facilitating Transfer

SST, like all training methods that take place away from the real situation, faces the problem of transfer of training, wherein learning that has taken place in the training environment must be transferred to the real environment. Thus in SST the skills learned during training must operate equally successfully in social interaction outside the training context. Research in this field has indicated that the two main difficulties with SST in clinical settings are in facilitating transfer, and maintaining improvements over time — in other words, the problems of generalisation and retention of skills. These problems should be borne in mind when deciding upon what techniques to employ during SST. The implementation of the following strategies can contribute towards improved transfer across situations and over time:

(1) The use of several members of staff, and other patients, during practicals. This allows the patient to gain experience in interacting with a range of other people in a controlled environment. The more people with whom the patient interacts successfully, the more will their confidence level improve, and the transfer of skills learned when interacting with one person to interactions with others will be facilitated. It is important, therefore, to present the patient with people of different age, sex and personality, as role-players during SST. There are, for example, different meanings and problems involved in eye contact with members of the opposite sex, as opposed to same-sex pairs. Such issues should be fully explored during training.

(2) The use of a wide range of practical exercises. All role-plays should be relevant to the setting in which the patient will later operate. Given this setting, it is possible to devise a number of problem situations that the patient will encounter (or has encountered) and use these as the basis for role-plays. At the same time, emphasis should be given to the elucidation of central principles of social interaction which can be used to handle various social encounters (listen to others, be assertive, etc.).

(3) Homework is a method for encouraging transfer during training. This is where the nurse sets the patient practical tasks to complete outside training sessions. The homework task is given at the end of one session and has to be completed before the beginning of the next session. The task set should relate to the behaviour under study, and should be within the capabilities of the patient. It should obviously relate to the situation in which the patient will be operating. Thus, the homework task may be to open a conversation with a stranger, have a meal in a cafe, or join in a group activity on the ward. The homework should be agreed as reasonable by the patient, and it is useful to formalise it by having a homework book in which the task is written and in which the patient notes his or her experiences in completing the task. The homework should then be discussed fully at the following session, and the patient

rewarded for success. Where success has not been attained, the reasons for failure should be investigated and the patient rewarded for trying. If necessary, role-play of the homework task can be enacted to provide further practice for the patient. By using this form of homework exercise, the patient is encouraged to transfer skills learned in training to the outside world.

(4) Practice can also take place outside the training situation, whereby the nurse can accompany the patient on a visit to a natural setting. This allows the nurse to observe and give feedback on the performance of the patient in a more realistic environment. Such visits can be time-consuming and may be difficult to organise, but they can be a potent learning experience for patients.

(5) Eventually the emphasis should be upon encouraging less reliance upon the nurse for feedback and developing in patients more confidence in their own ability to handle social situations. This, in effect, means a certain degree of cognitive restructuring on the part of the patients during SST. The nurse should facilitate this process by having patients discuss their thoughts and feelings concerning all practical tasks and helping patients to think things out for themselves. This will involve the use of open questions during discussions of practicals (e.g. 'What were you thinking about at that time?' 'If he had not answered what would you have done?' 'How do you think she felt about that?') to encourage the self-monitoring capacity of the patient. Self-monitoring refers to the ability of the person to monitor their own behaviour and take corrective action if necessary (e.g. 'I'm being left out of this discussion — I must get back into it', 'He doesn't seem to understand, I'd better explain that again'). As explained in Chapter 4, with practice such cognitive processes become subconscious, but during skill learning they should be consciously employed. The patient should also develop the capacity to monitor their feelings and rationalise these (e.g. 'I'm getting anxious about this, but there is really nothing to it': 'He doesn't seem to like me, but that's OK, I won't worry too much about it'). As well as self-monitoring, the process of self-reinforcement should be developed in patients, whereby the patient does not depend upon reward from the nurse, but can function adequately by reinforcing himself (e.g. 'I handled that well', 'I listened care-

fully to him', 'That was a good discussion'). Both self-monitoring and self-reinforcement encourage the patient to operate independently.

(6) The use of follow-up (or 'booster') sessions some time after termination of the SST programme can serve to maintain skill improvements. There will inevitably be some detriment in the level of skills, which tend to atrophy once training ceases, but this can be retarded by organising refresher sessions. During these refreshers attention should be given to those situations in which the patient still finds difficulty.

Overview

This chapter has been concerned with the core elements of SST. It will be realised that the methods used in the training of social skills are, in a sense, nothing new. The methods of training used in the analysis and training of motor skills have now been applied to the training of social skills in terms of sensitisation, modelling, practice and feedback. The popularity and apparent success of this approach are due in part to this familiarity, and in part to the opportunity it offers to improve the social performance and mental health of a large number of patients. All the components discussed in this chapter are of vital import to the successful operation of SST. Assessment of patients is crucial at the outset, to ascertain the nature and extent of skill deficits. Once these have been identified, attention needs to be given to the training methods employed to attempt to overcome them. Finally, the issues of generalisation and retention of skills should always be uppermost in the mind of the nurse, to ensure the overall success of SST.

6 IMPLEMENTING AN SST PROGRAMME

Each step of an SST programme is of equal importance; just as inaccurate and inappropriate assessment and planning can lead to failure, so too can improper implementation. In many instances, the actual implementation can in fact be the most difficult stage, requiring much time and tolerance on the part of both the nurse and the patient. Failure at this advanced stage can be detrimental to all involved. Patients with heightened expectations can be deflated and discouraged, whilst staff can lose their enthusiasm for carrying out the treatment. Meticulous execution of SST programmes is therefore imperative if any degree of success is to be achieved. This chapter builds on the previous, exploring the practicalities of implementing an SST programme within a psychiatric nursing context. Issues examined include: group and individual approaches to SST; knowledge of and attitudes to SST; differences in approach and objectives with long-stay as opposed to short-stay patients; availability of SST resources; contracts in treatment; ethical issues and finally evaluation of SST. Suggestions are offered throughout the chapter on how to circumvent possible problems that may arise when implementing an SST programme.

Group and Individual Approaches to SST

When implementing an SST programme, the psychiatric nurse will be confronted with many realities that can often impede and limit the success of the programme. Manpower resources, for instance, may dictate the amount of time a nurse can spend with individual patients. It would be both unrealistic and impractical to employ individual SST programmes in situations where the nurse-patient ratio is unsuitable. Conversely, individual SST programmes may be the only solution with certain psychiatric patients, irrespective of nurse-patient ratios. Compromise, therefore, may have to be agreed upon.

The use of group and individual SST approaches are dependent on several factors, with each approach having its own particular advantages and disadvantages. Cognisance must be taken of the following factors when determining what type of SST approach should be used.

(1) The nurse-patient ratio, as stated earlier, may influence the type of SST approach used. It is obviously more economical in terms of time for a nurse to work with a group as opposed to one individual patient. Strictly speaking, however, ratios should not be a criterion for deciding what type of SST approach is used. Rather, selection should be determined by the suitability of the approach for a particular patient.

(2) The type of patient may also determine the type of SST approach employed. Some patients, as suggested by Trower et al (1978), may be too disturbed or regressed for group sessions, while others may become too highly anxious when asked to function within a group setting. Such patients would warrant more prolonged attention and would perhaps respond more favourably to an individual SST programme.

(3) When a group SST approach is decided upon, careful thought must be given to the types of patient selected. Opinions differ, however, as to what criteria should be used to determine group participants. Patients, for example, may be grouped according to age, intelligence, diagnosis or even social background. Wilkinson and Canter (1983) suggest that no such criteria should be used, but recognise that 'patients with some characteristics in common might feel that other group members have a better understanding of their difficulties and can be more supportive'. They add that a mix of patients may be advantageous in that it gives a variety of models, provides partners for role play and allows for more comprehensive feedback. Conversely Trower et al (1978) do suggest criteria for selecting patients for SST groups, namely: patients with observable skill deficits (i.e. socially inadequate); and patients with competence in skills but whose performance is disrupted by anxiety. Selecting patients for group SST may therefore be difficult and only careful evaluation of the patient's performance during group work will enable the nurse to determine more fully the patient's suitability.

(4) When conducting group SST the nurse must carefully control the number within the group. Most trainers recommend group sizes comprising of between six to twelve patients. Larger groups are often impractical since patients may adopt a more

passive role, and not participate as much as they should. The smaller the group, therefore, the more the patient will be compelled to get involved.

(5) In certain cases both group and individual SST programmes may be used simultaneously. Patients, in addition to working within groups, may need extra individual attention for specific problems. Others who are so disturbed or regressed may require many individual sessions before being introduced to the group. Either way, the approaches should not be seen as separate entities but rather as training that can operate concurrently.

In addition to the above, the nurse must also be aware of the consequences of the techniques employed. Group SST can be a useful approach for several reasons:

(1) By involving the patient in an SST group, the nurse is providing a ready-made social learning situation. Such situations tend to be less simulated than individual sessions and allow the patient to practise new skills in a relaxed and accepting environment.

(2) Training models as suggested in the previous chapter are very important. Groups enable a variety of models to be used and so increase the likelihood that the patient will at least identify with one or more of the models used. Fellow patients used as models in group situations are also more likely to portray problems similar to those faced by the patient. Conversely, nurses who role model in individual SST programmes may be seen as 'too good' and as a consequence the patient has difficulty identifying with them. Caution must be taken with negative models. Too frequent exposure to and/or inadequate explanation of negative behaviour could result in inappropriate skills being learned.

(3) Patients can act not only as models but also as a source of encouragement. A patient commencing a group SST programme may be motivated through observing and talking to fellow patients with similar problems who have improved as a result of training. Such an exercise may also enable patients to see their own deficits more clearly.

(4) It is imperative that the skills learned carry over into everyday, real-life social situations (i.e. generalise). Group SST can help

facilitate this generalisation, as suggested by Spence (1980), by affording patients a variety of individuals as models rather than one trainer alone. This allows the patient to interact with others from different backgrounds (i.e. with a variety of age, intelligence, sex etc.). Thus the patient can gradually build up a degree of confidence and competence in dealing with different social situations, and this, in turn, will assist in the generalisation of skills acquired during SST.

(5) Feedback on a patient's performance by fellow patients can be a potent source of social reinforcement. If used appropriately it may not only serve to enhance further participation but can also encourage patients to observe and analyse social interactions both critically and constructively.

(6) Having been introduced to one another during group work, patients may come together outside formal SST sessions to practise the skills acquired. This may either be a spontaneous exercise or alternatively be imposed in the form of homework. Either way, knowledge of one another through group work can facilitate practice at a later stage.

In contrast to group SST, individual training approaches may in certain cases be more applicable for a number of reasons:

Flexibility

Individual programmes can be carefully compiled to suit the specific needs of the patient. This may entail dealing with problems that are not commonly encountered in a group situation. Such flexibility also enables the pace of the programme to be altered in order to suit the patient's rate of progress.

Intensity

In certain situations patients may require intensive training. Individual SST programmes enable the nurse to spend more time with the patient, therefore allowing for a greater concentration of effort. This hopefully would lead to more rapid progress being made by the patient.

Types of Patient

Some patients, as stated earlier, may prove too disruptive or withdrawn for group situations. This may result in their either upsetting the therapeutic nature of the group or refusing to participate.

Either way such individuals may initially require individual attention before progressing to group settings.

More Practice

Unlike group programmes, individual sessions allow the patient to practise their skills over a long period. This allows for quicker acquisition of the skill.

Some of the advantages of each training approach are summarized in Figure 6.1. The nurse may find it difficult at times to decide which SST approach should be used. It is perhaps only after one approach has been employed that the nurse will more accurately ascertain its suitability. Determining the suitability of either group or individual SST can be summarised in the words of Eisler and Frederiksen (1980), who in comparing both formats concluded 'in choosing between an individual or group format, the trainer must be mindful of the nature of the client's skill deficits. If the clients have similar backgrounds and show similar skill deficits, it is probably wise to use a group format. If on the other hand, the clients have a variety of dissimilar backgrounds and differing skill deficits, an individual format is indicated.'

Knowledge of and Attitudes to SST

Only when an SST programme has actually been implemented and evaluated can the nurse fully appreciate the inherent problems in

Figure 6.1: Some Advantages of Individual and Group SST Approaches

Individual SST	Group SST
Can deal with specific patient needs	Is more cost-effective
Has inherent flexibility	Provides ready made social learning situation
Can be paced to suit patients' needs	Offers a variety of models
Requires greater intensity of effort	Affords patient encouragement from fellow patients
Allows for more practice	Facilitates transfer

employing such an approach. Obviously, there are occasional problems thrown up by the patient and the appropriateness of the treatment programme. In addition to these, however, when implementing an SST regime the nurse will periodically encounter certain extraneous hurdles which are sometimes of their own making and sometimes outside their control. Many of these hurdles or problems arise within or stem from other staff. It is perhaps salutary at this point, therefore, to take a brief, realistic look at some of the problems the nurse will encounter when implementing an SST programme.

Little research has been carried out into nursing staff knowledge of and attitudes to SST. Much of the information therefore is based upon the writers' own experiences, gained as course tutors when working with post-basic students. The students drawn from six psychiatric hospitals undertook, as part of course criteria, SST within their own clinical setting. Feedback was obtained via both formal instrumentation and informal discussion and a number of points emerged:

(1) Students suggested that they had insufficient knowledge to implement an SST programme properly. They suggested that a more solid knowledge base would be necessary for the nurse to use this form of training confidently and competently. One must concede that nurse education has, until recently, fallen short in properly preparing and orientating nurses towards this form of social treatment. Briggs and Wright (1982) echo this sentiment when they suggest that 'while courses on personal effectiveness training for nurses have increased in America, British students are inadequately prepared for the social role in nursing. Introductory courses offer no training or development of these skills.' Recent advances, however, have been made. With the new training syllabus, nurses will be gradually introduced to the concept throughout their training.

(2) The term SST appeared to have different meanings, not only between nursing staff but also within other disciplines. Many nursing personnel, for example, defined social skills as 'coping' or 'daily living' skills. Conversely, others believed them to be essentially interactional skills, comprising such elements as listening, questioning, reinforcement and nonverbal communication. Since this ambiguity has already been fully discussed in Chapter 2 it will perhaps suffice here to add that it is impera-

tive that all staff have a common understanding of the concept. Differences in perceptions can only lead to confusion and failure. Proper education regarding SST, therefore, via inservice and post-basic training, with nursing personnel actively seeking out relevant material, is essential.

(3) Ward staff's feelings about, and subsequent behaviour towards, SST varied markedly, ranging from full co-operation to outright opposition. Reasons for this opposition were not always explicit, but some were nevertheless clearly defined. Firstly, the age-old arguments were voiced, e.g. 'We've tried that before and it didn't work' 'It's a waste of time, that patient will never improve'. Secondly, some recognised the long-term benefits of the approach but suggested that the nurse spent too much time with one or more of the patients to the detriment of others. Thirdly, some staff openly admitted that they knew very little about the concept and therefore were reluctant to get involved.

Undoubtedly many of these problems will be difficult to circumvent, no matter how the subject is broached. In order to minimise their effects, the nurse must consider very closely the way in which the concept is introduced; all too often such problems can arise if the concept is introduced inappropriately. Consider the following situation for example:

A patient suffering from chronic schizophrenia has been nursed within a particular ward for six years. A new member of nursing staff decides that the patient would benefit from SST, and so following brief consultation with the ward manager, attempts to implement a programme.

An extreme example perhaps — or is it? There are many implications of adopting such an approach. Apart from the serious ethical implications of not involving the patient in the treatment regime, what might other staff feel, particularly those who were not involved initially? A natural reaction might be not to get involved, especially if one's contribution was not valued in the beginning. Alternatively, some nursing staff might see it as a slight on the care they have been delivering over the last six years. Either way, the example emphasises the need for SST programmes to be introduced diplomatically. Care must be taken to involve and value all staff contributions, remembering that staff are more likely to participate if they themselves have been involved in the initial stages of the programming.

(4) There was a significant lack of multidiscipline teamwork when implementing SST programmes. This may have arisen as a result of several factors. Obviously, like their nursing colleagues, other disciplines like to be informed and involved throughout programming. In some circumstances, however, other disciplines refused to participate because they saw SST as being their responsibility. Nurses, therefore, were seen to be encroaching upon their roles. This occasionally leads to friction, even resentment, between the 'caring' parties involved. Unfortunately, this inter-discipline rivalry can ultimately affect the care delivered, with the patient being caught in the middle. Overcoming such a problem may prove difficult. Nurses must refrain from considering themselves in competition with others, but rather should attempt to engender a multidiscipline team spirit and enthusiasm. Responsibility falls also with other disciplines in creating such an environment. All concerned in providing patient care must realise the potential of a multidiscipline approach, not forgetting they are all working towards a common goal.

(5) As a result of the problems mentioned above, many SST programmes failed to be fully implemented (due to lack of knowledge, support etc.). This in turn had repercussions for the nurse implementing the programme, the patient or patients involved and for other staff. The nurse trainer, because of lack of success and support, became disenchanted with the treatment, while the patient or patient's hopes were dashed. Failure also helped to substantiate the negative views of some staff that the treatment was a waste of time and effort.

In using SST therefore, the nurse trainer must ensure that training will be fully implemented according to the treatment plan. Any factor that might interfere with the treatment regime should be fully investigated prior to commencing training, and where possible the effects rectified or minimised. The inability to do so may necessitate the use of other more suitable treatment approaches.

(6) Many SST programmes failed because the initial assessment was often found to be limited and subjective. In such cases the nurse trainer frequently failed to include other staff and

patients in treatment programming. Therefore, restricted contributions from others resulted in assessments and evaluations being based solely on the nurse trainer's own observations.

(7) Finally, there were certain ethical implications in implementing such SST programmes. Is it ethically right, for example, to undertake a programme with the knowledge that the nurse trainer will be moved prior to its full implementation? Is it acceptable to implement a programme without first securing some form of patient agreement or contract? SST must be undertaken with the sole objective of helping the patient, and any circumstance that may impede that objective *must* be resolved before embarking on the programme.

In conclusion, the nurse may encounter numerous problems when implementing an SST programme. These may be circumvented, firstly, by ensuring that nurses possess the necessary clinical skills to enable them to undertake the training competently. Such skills, as suggested by Faulkner (1985), must become an integral part of all curricula for nurses, with tutors themselves possessing the skills to teach by experiential methods. Secondly, when implementing an SST programme the nurse must recognise the importance of the roles of nursing colleagues, other disciplines and the patients involved. Neglecting to do so will invariably result in failure of the SST programme.

Short and Long-term Patients

No two patients can be considered the same when designing and implementing an SST programme. Each will have their unique needs and idiosyncrasies which require and demand individual attention. Such individualised treatment may, for instance, necessitate specific assessment techniques to be used, or perhaps a particular training method. Nowhere, however, are these differences more obvious than between short- and long-term patients. In dealing with such categories of patients the nurse will be confronted with not only a wide variety of social skill deficits but also different extraneous factors that may influence the course of training. It is perhaps salutary at this point, therefore, to reiterate the types of social skill deficit that may be encountered, highlighting some of the differences which may arise when implementing an SST programme.

Deficit Differences

A quite significant variation in social skill deficits exists within the psychiatrically ill population. As discussed in Chapter 2 (Figure 2.3) deficits may range from anomalies in the daily living components at the bottom of the hierarchy through to problems in larger social skill elements such as making friends, dating or being interviewed. Such a range is typically reflected in long-stay patients, presenting primarily with anomalies in daily living skills, and short-term patients with deficits further up the hierarchy. Although nurses must appreciate the relationship between the various skills when compiling and implementing training, they must also recognise the significant differences that exist and how they in turn may effect programming. The nurse, for example, must appreciate the necessity for meeting the patient's social skill deficits in terms of priority. Therefore, deficits at the base of the hierarchy must be fully ameliorated before tackling other social skill components higher up. Differences, however, in the deficits encountered between the various categories of patients are also of major significance to the nurse, especially when contemplating SST for long-stay patients. Such significant areas include:

Contract Formation.   Forming a genuine contract with long-stay patients may, at times, be problematic. The patient's ability to comprehend fully what the treatment is about may be impaired for a variety of reasons. (These reasons will be explored in the section on contracts and so will not be discussed here). Conversely, the patient may be able to understand but may not have the necessary motivation to participate in the training. It must be remembered that in addition to primary psychiatric symptoms, many of the long-stay population also display the effects of institutionalisation and as a result become rather apathetic about their treatment. SST without proper contract formation must be considered inappropriate.

Relevant Literature.   As already suggested many of the deficits encountered in the long-stay population fall within the 'daily living skill' sector. Much of the SST literature concentrates on skills higher up the hierarchy, therefore supportive reading material may not be so readily available. Nevertheless, there is an increasing awareness that such techniques can be applied to enhance these basic social skills (Westland, 1980; Van Den Pol et al, 1981).

SST Approaches. The SST approaches used with long-stay patients may differ for several reasons. Firstly, many patients will require training on an individual basis. This may be due to the chronic nature of the deficits where the patients require intense and prolonged training. Secondly, it may not always be possible to group patients in long-stay areas. Deficits can range so markedly that it is often difficult to select suitable patients. In grouping, the nurse must ensure that suitable positive models are available, but inappropriate models are all too readily available in such areas, a factor that possibly contributes to the patient's deficits in the first place. Thirdly, training objectives may have to be broken down into smaller sub-objectives, which will assist the patient to understand more fully what is to be achieved. Sub-objectives may also be useful where progress is slow, in reinforcing the patient (i.e. rewarding as each small step is accomplished).

Generalisation. Generalisation of skills may be particularly difficult for long-stay patients. Many of these patients live in environments where the opportunities to practise skills acquired are limited. In addition, as suggested earlier, such environments contain many inappropriate models who could quickly undo everything that has been achieved. Restrictions in the use of a variety of models (i.e. through group work) may also impede the transfer of skills by not affording the patient the opportunity to interact with several different people or groups. Finally long-stay patients, because of their limited contact with people outside their immediate environment, will have problems in addition to those of generalising the skills learned. Imagine, for example, the patient who has not left hospital for several years. If people without social skill deficits can have difficulty coping with new situations, what must it be like for patients with problems in interacting? The nurse must recognise this when undertaking SST and attempt to make use of real-life situations when and where possible, in order to aid generalisation.

SST Resources

To be successful SST must, like other forms of treatment, have certain resources at its disposal. Such resources include any 'ingredients' (i.e. people, facilities, materials and equipment) that are needed to run SST effectively. The nurse may find the following suggestions helpful when considering the use of resources in SST:

(1) The size of the room required will depend upon the type of SST approach used. A one-to-one format, for example, will require less accommodation than group training. Either way, patients should be afforded sufficient space to move around freely if need be. This helps to create a more relaxed and congenial atmosphere and is essential if role-play techniques are to be used.

(2) Such environments must include appropriate 'props' to assist in role-play exercises. In the simulation of a shopping situation, for example, the use of a table and till may be helpful.

(3) In group situations the nurse should ensure that all patients have similar chairs and spacing. Chairs should be placed in a circular fashion so that all group members feel equal and can see and hear everyone else.

(4) Teaching aids (e.g. blackboard, flipchart, or overhead projector) should be used wherever possible. These are useful if the nurse wants to clarify or emphasise certain points.

(5) Privacy and confidentiality are of paramount importance. Sessions therefore should run uninterrupted and unobserved; observation (e.g. via a viewing window) may only take place following the patient's permission.

(6) An additional trainer may be used where the demands of a group are too great for one nurse. The second nurse may also be used to operate the audio-visual equipment.

(7) The use of video playback facilities has already been fully discussed in the previous chapter. When these are used, it is helpful if the camera can be made as inconspicuous as possible so as to minimise distractions and enable the patient to become less aware of being video-taped.

(8) Finally, resources outside the immediate hospital setting may also be used. In some instances it may be necessary to follow the training sessions with *in situ* training (i.e. moving from a simulated exercise to a real-life setting). For example, the

patient who has difficulty shopping may (following SST exercises on the ward) go out shopping with the nurse. Such resources must be carefully assessed by the nurse before *in situ* training, in order to ensure suitability.

Nurse-patient Contracts

Interest in nurse-patient contracting has gained momentum over the past 10 years (Langford, 1972; Gustafson, 1977; Coombe et al, 1981). Although an integral part of SST, it is nevertheless a relatively new concept to nursing and so perhaps warrants further discussion.

The process of contracting between nurses and clients, as suggested by Loomis (1985), is based on several assumptions. The first and most important of these is that patients have the right to make decisions regarding their own health care. A second and related assumption is that nurses are responsible professionals, capable of negotiating with patients for the care they will provide. Contracting in SST may initially place the nurse in an unfamiliar situation. Where she previously dictated the treatments she must now come together with the patient and seek agreement about goals and have a clear understanding of the responsibilities of each. This could also prove difficult for the patient. As suggested by Loomis (1985), many 'come from a long history of being passive recipients of nursing and health care interventions, and therefore have little experience with the process of negotiating for their needs with a provider of care'. Not only therefore, may both parties have to contend with the inherent problems of agreeing, they must also overcome the trauma of actually being involved in the contracting process.

Contracting Process

There are certain points that the nurse must bear in mind when formulating SST contracts:

(1) Information given to the patient must, as suggested by Eisler and Frederiksen (1980), be complete, truthful and fully understood. Patients, for example, may agree to participate in treatment while not fully understanding what it is about. The patient may perhaps be too frightened, or may even believe he

has no right, to question. Conversely, when explaining, nurses may take too much for granted and fail to ensure that the patient fully comprehends what is going on. Either way, time spent openly discussing what the programme entails is time well spent, since such preparation can only help to enhance both understanding and participation. In addition, this explanatory session can also be useful in allaying patient fears. Knowing what is to happen, and why, can be extremely useful in reducing anxieties often associated with new treatments.

(2) Although related to the above point, truthfulness and openness is worthy of singular recognition. In addition to seeking agreement during contracting, the nurse through being truthful and open can build up a trusting and meaningful rapport with the patient. This is of paramount importance and can often determine the success or failure of SST.

(3) The patient must freely consent to participate in the described training programme. Never under any circumstances must the nurse or others attempt to pressurise the patient into getting involved. Frequently, however, in their unbounding enthusiasm to help those within their care, psychiatric nurses fail to recognise that not all patients want to change. Thus although staff may identify obvious social skill deficits in a patient and wish to undertake an SST programme, if the patient is not properly motivated to get involved or does not consider his deficits to be problems, then the suitability of SST must be questioned.

(4) Care must be taken when deciding upon what type of contract (i.e. verbal or written) should be used. Some patients may see a written statement as being too formal and 'legal' and this may even frighten the patient. Conversely, a verbal contract may be subject to memory variations and distortions. The decision therefore, differs from patient to patient and may only be determined through observations and actual discussion with the patient. Occasionally it may be recognised, following implementation of the programme, that a particular type of contract is unsuitable. The patient, for instance, who has difficulty retaining information may benefit from a written as opposed to a verbal contract. It must also be remembered that contracts should be re-negotiable, affording a degree of flexibility after evaluation. In this way, the patient who previously consented to be video-taped, should be allowed the freedom

to re-consider and discuss his decision.

(5) The written contract example given in Chapter 5 (Figure 5.7) seeks to obtain general permission and commitment from the patient. In addition, it may also be helpful to include the short- and long-term objectives of the programme. By so doing, more specific patient commitment can be obtained (i.e. the patient must undertake a particular task by a certain date). Such a breakdown affords the patient feedback on how well he is progressing, which can in turn be reinforcing as each step is accomplished.

(6) Some patients, as stated in Chapter 2, may not be suitable for SST, principally because they are unable to negotiate a meaningful contract. This may be due to a variety of reasons. For instance, the patient with distorted thinking processes and impairment of concentration may find it difficult to comprehend what the treatment is about. Alternatively, some patients may not have the cognitive abilities to grasp fully what is being explained. Failure to negotiate the contract at the very outset necessitates discontinuation of the approach.

(7) When compiling contract objectives it is imperative that they are realistic, explicit and obtainable. Failure to ensure this can result in unclear expectations, unmet goals and anxiety and frustration in both the patient and the nurse trainer.

(8) When working within group situations, contracts can remain on an individual basis but with certain added group agreements. Group members can discuss and agree upon the actual mechanics of running the group (e.g. punctuality and schedules).

In conclusion, contract formation is probably the most important single aspect in SST. The patient's commitment and full participation are essential in determining the success of training. The nurse must, therefore, ensure that adequate time and deliberation are given to this important process.

Ethical Issues

As with any programme that attempts to effect behaviour change in patients, there are a number of ethical issues that need to be borne in mind when designing and implementing SST programmes. Some of these have already been mentioned, but this is such an important aspect of training that we do not apologise for emphasising them again. The main ethical issues involved are as below.

Have Nurses the Right to Attempt to Change Overtly the Behaviour of Patients?

This issue is fundamental to the whole concept of remedial SST, which is geared specifically towards direct behavioural intervention. The question can be answered in the affirmative. SST programmes are not entered into lightly, but are comprehensively discussed by the entire multidiscipline team. Patients are volunteers in SST, are told exactly what is involved in this form of training, agree the goals which are set, and enter into a contract of some form with the nurse trainer. Providing that this degree of patient consent is obtained, SST is justifiable. The nurse and patient become trainer and trainee respectively; they form a training partnership, and the emphasis is more upon education than treatment. This level of commitment must be reciprocal, with the nurse being convinced of the worth of both the patient and the programme. Once a programme has been entered into, it should be completed by the nurse, as their part of the contract. If there are any difficulties about not being able to complete the programme, the nurse must either make these explicit at the outset, or, more probably, not enter into a training commitment. Such an open approach is, in fact, more ethical than traditional medical approaches where the patient is often totally unaware of decisions taken about him or her, or the nature of treatment being administered. Providing, therefore, that the goals of SST are to benefit the patient (and not the institution), this is ethically acceptable. It should be remembered that, while the results of SST will generally be of value both to the patient and the hospital, the latter benefits should be incidental. It would not be acceptable to run SST programmes designed to facilitate the smooth running of the hospital by, for example, encouraging patient conformity or submissiveness.

Does SST Teach Patients How to Manipulate Others?

In one sense this is true, in that following training patients should be able to implement a number of behaviours that can be employed to influence others. But these are behaviours that the 'normal' population are already using, and which, for some reason, patients have not acquired skill in implementing successfully. Another ethical question here is whether it is justifiable for some people to be denied access to information, knowledge or skill that is already widely available. Those who believe in SST as a valid form of remediation would argue that it is not justifiable to deny access to such an important dimension as the ability to communicate successfully with other people. There is always the danger that some patients will use their new skills malevolently, but this does not negate the validity of the training process. Just because some individuals write obscene graffiti on walls, or send poison pen letters to others, does not mean that it is unethical to teach people how to write! The heightened awareness and increased skill resulting from SST will be gratefully received by the vast majority of patients, who will use this knowledge in a meaningful and constructive fashion.

Are there Dangers in Recording a Patient's Behaviour on Videotape?

As has already been pointed out, there are indeed dangers in video-recording the behaviour of patients during SST. The patient should give full consent to allowing this to take place, should be informed in advance of some of the possible reactions they may experience, should be able to withdraw at any time from video-recording, and should never suffer unduly from being exposed to video feedback. Patients should always be fully aware of when they are being recorded, and no subterfuge should be entered into. Strict control of all video tapes collected during training is essential, and they should be erased as soon as possible after practicals. Where a tape is to be kept for any reason, or is to be used for research or teaching purposes, explicit written permission must be obtained from all those involved on the tape. If a good role-play is recorded during SST and it is felt that this could serve as a useful positive model exemplar for other patients, then this should be fully explained to the actors, and their written permission for its use sought. Under no circumstances should a role-play involving patients be used as a negative model exemplar. The patient should have confidence in the ability of the nurse to refuse access to tapes to anyone other than those directly involved in the training programme. In other words, the patient must be able to trust both the nurse, and the system of video-recording.

Do SST Programmes Destroy Individuality and Produce Uniformity of Behaviour?

This argument is usually put forward by socially skilled individuals! The suggestion here is that SST teaches a fixed set of behavioural responses which will eventually end up producing a series of robot-like humans. Furthermore, by social skills being taught, social interaction will lose its natural beauty and become artificial and stilted. Everyone will become so aware of their own actions and the actions and reactions of others that this knowledge will inhibit their natural behaviour. However, this is rather like saying that by teaching everyone to talk, we will all eventually end up saying exactly the same things. Individual differences will always influence the ways in which people behave socially. Personality, home background, attitudes and values, will invariably affect an individual's goals in any given situation, and this in turn will affect behaviour. There is absolutely no evidence to suggest that after SST everyone will conform to a set pattern of behaviour in a given situation. What SST does is to attempt to extend the repertoire of behavioural alternatives open to patients, thereby increasing their freedom of expression. In addition, by adopting the nursing process philosophy, the goals of remedial SST should be individualised, rather than pre-determined, and should be geared to meet the particular needs of each patient.

Does SST Ignore Problems of Class and Culture?

This issue is related in some respects to the previous one, and it is a danger in SST. The nurse should always take account of the environment within which the patient will operate, and be aware of the behaviourally acceptable patterns within that environment. For example, it is counterproductive and invalid to attempt to inculcate middle-class behaviours in working class patients. Similarly, care must be taken when training patients from ethnic minority groups. Differences in eye-contact patterns have been found between West Indians and white males in England, in that the former group look at a partner more while speaking and less while listening than the latter group, and it would be inappropriate to teach white gaze patterns to a West Indian male. The concept of 'cultural expertise' (Ivey and Authier, 1978) should be given emphasis in this context. This refers to the ability of an individual to communicate effectively with a maximum number of individuals in any given cultural setting. Thus, patients who will interact with people from a different ethnic or class background should be given an awareness of the different behavioural responses that predominate. The problem, especially for nurses working in large urban conurbations, is in identifying these patterns across subcultures. This may involve extensive observation of, and discussion with, ethnic minorities. Certainly, when dealing with patients, no one set of behaviour patterns should be taken as given.

Evaluation of SST

In order to assess the effectiveness of SST, it is necessary to conduct some form of evaluation of the training programme that has been implemented. This provides the nurse with vital feedback regarding the extent to which the objectives have been achieved and whether, and in what ways, elements of the programme need to be altered. The evaluation of SST can be more or less rigorous and sophisticated, depending upon the time, resources and expertise available. In reality, practical problems often inhibit the pursuit of experimentally sophisticated evaluation. Quite often there will be no back-up, in terms of research staff, to assist in the operation of such an evaluation, or little emphasis will be placed upon sophisticated research by the agency within which the nurse functions. The nurse may have a heavy workload and hence very little time to devote to research. Other problems here include the difficulty in obtaining a comparable control group (agency policy may even discourage this) against which to evaluate the SST group, and the lack of valid instruments with which to measure the often very specific goals of training.

Those methods that have been used initially to assess the patient can, and should, be used to evaluate the patient following SST. Thus, the procedures described in Chapter 5 are all relevant as evaluation methods. The patient can be interviewed post-training about the extent to which SST has alleviated the problems originally identified, and can be questioned about his or her own reactions to the training itself. This type of information can also be gleaned from questionnaires administered to patients following training, in which they are asked specifically about their SST experience, and elements thereof. In this way, information can be gathered about the perceived influence of the trainers, other patients, CCTV, role-plays and so on. Specific feedback can also be obtained from other members of staff who may be asked to fill in the same (or a slightly adjusted version) questionnaire that they completed pre-SST (see Figure 5.1).

Self-report measures can also provide a useful source of data concerning how SST has directly influenced the patient. Do they view themselves more positively after training? Has their self-esteem improved? Do they report fewer problems than before? However, in many respects the acid test of the effectiveness of SST is whether they have improved in terms of their behavioural performance. In theory, this should be measured *in vivo*, that is when the patient is interacting in his or her natural environment. In practice, this can cause both logistical and ethical problems. Where should the patient be observed, and by whom? On how many occasions should the patient be observed? Should the patient be told that he will be observed? If so, will this interfere with his behaviour? As a result, role-play is often used as a compromise, despite the obvious difficulties in generalising from behaviour during role-play to behaviour in the natural environment. One advantage of it is that it can be video-recorded for detailed behaviour analysis. Ratings of the patient can be made and behaviour counts taken, to determine the exact effects of SST.

As wide a variety as possible of these methods should be used to provide the maximum degree of feedback on the programme, and how it has influenced the patient's thoughts, feelings and behaviour. Where homework assignments have been given and a homework book used, it is interesting to examine this and chart the degree to which the patient's ability to use self-monitoring and self-reinforcement techniques have developed during the programme. These are the main methods available to the nurse involved in SST who wishes to obtain some indication regarding the effects of training upon patients.

Where the nurse is working as a member of a team involved in SST, then it may be more feasible to attempt an in-depth evaluation of the effects of training. Where the behaviour of patients involved in SST can be compared with a matched control group, greater confidence can be placed in attributing any post-training gains that the SST group display over the control group to the training programme itself. In practice, a control group cannot always be employed, and in such instances, three main types of experimental design are employed in SST.

Pre-post Training Comparison

As the name suggests, this involves obtaining measures of patients pre-SST and again post-SST and assessing the extent of change that has taken place. This is the simplest and most easily implemented design, since measures are taken on only two occasions. There is a range of statistical tests available for comparing matched pairs of subjects on two occasions, so with group SST programmes the level of significance of objective data can be determined. With individual SST, a direct comparison can be made, but no indication can be obtained regarding level of significance. However, in neither case can any changes that occur be attributed directly to SST since they may have been caused by other factors, such as events outside the training environment or developmental changes in patients that would have occurred regardless of SST. Nevertheless, this type of design does provide basic, and valuable, information for evaluating SST.

Time Series Analysis

This is an extension of the pre-post training analysis to take account of the influence of repeated practice as a possible cause of change during SST. Time series analysis basically consists of collecting measures on aspects of the patient on a number of occasions pre-training and on a number of occasions post-training, such as:

W1   W2   W3   W4   W5   T6   T7   T8   T9   T10   T11
T12   T13   T14   T15   W16   W17   W18   W19   W20

Here the same measures are taken once a week 'W' for 5 weeks before training; this is followed by 10 training weeks 'T'; and then the same measures are taken once a week for 5 weeks following training. In essence, this method involves a number of pre-tests and a number of post-tests. It is, therefore, more difficult to utilise and more time-consuming to carry out. It has the advantage of ensuring that change is not caused by practice alone since this would emerge from W1 to W5 and from W16 to W20, and it can be used with single subjects to determine the significant level of change (although this requires a large number of observations). There remains the problem that, in the absence of a control group, change could be attributed directly to the training programme.

Multiple Baseline Analysis

This form of experimental design has become widely used in research into remedial SST, since it overcomes the problem of lack of control group and provides a method whereby change can be attributed to the training intervention. It involves consistently measuring a number of behaviours on a number of occasions during SST. The behaviours are measured, usually on three occasions, prior to SST, and this represents the initial baseline data. Then each behaviour is introduced for training purposes on separate weeks. If training is successful, then behaviour change should occur only on the week in which the behaviour is introduced (see Figure 6.2), with no change occurring on other behaviours. In this way, behaviour change can be directly linked to training, by comparing the baseline measurements for each behaviour against the measurement for that behaviour in the first session in which it is introduced during SST. Thus, from Figure 6.2, it can be seen that during the baseline assessment, this patient never engaged in eye contact, but following the introduction and practice of this topic in SST, he increased gaze duration to 35 seconds. Similarly, during baseline assessment, the patient generally only smiled once, but when this topic was introduced in SST he increased his number of smiles to 10. As can be seen, this method requires a number of measurements over a period of time and can therefore be time-consuming. It does, however, offer a greater degree of confidence in relating changes in patients to their SST experience.

Overview

Some of the practicalities of implementing an SST programme within a psychiatric nursing context have been discussed in this chapter. It will be apparent from this brief review that successful implementation depends not merely on relating theory to practice but also on the nurse's ability to circumvent the many problems that may arise. It is not always possible to legislate for such problems when planning, so the nurse must display great diplomacy and fortitude when broaching the subject.

In introducing SST as a form of remediation treatment, therefore, the nurse must primarily use his or her own social skills effectively in order to gain not only the patient's full co-operation

Figure 6.2: Example of Multiple Baseline Approach

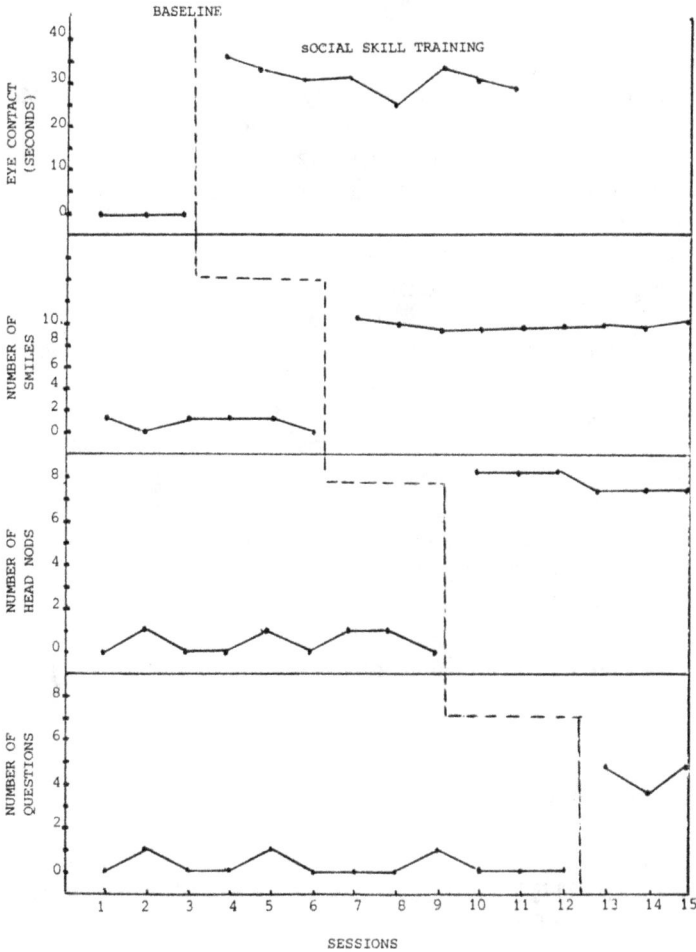

but also that of nursing colleagues and fellow disciplines. The nurse should also be aware of a number of other issues in SST, including group and individual approaches with short- and long-term patients; contract formation; ethical concerns; and methods for evaluating the effectiveness of programmes. All of these issues need to be considered by the nurse when planning and implementing SST.

7 CORE SOCIAL SKILLS

This chapter is concerned with an analysis of what we have termed 'core' social skills, because of their importance in establishing relationships. We have included three skill areas in this category namely: nonverbal communication, self-disclosure, and greetings and partings.

Nonverbal communication is an important area of study, given that it is present in various forms in every interaction between two people. Indeed all of the other skills discussed in this chapter, and in Chapters 8 and 9, contain nonverbal elements, so an understanding of the main facets of this channel will facilitate an examination of the remaining skills. Self-disclosure is also a crucial aspect of interpersonal interaction, especially in the early stages of relationship development when information about self is given and received by both people. The final area of study in this chapter concerns the skills of meeting people, and closing interactions satisfactorily. Such greetings and partings are of vital import both in our everyday conversations with friends or acquaintances and when meeting people for the first time. Thus, these three skill areas play a significant part in the process of interpersonal communication.

Nonverbal Communication

This area of study has received a vast amount of attention over the past 20 years. This interest has been stimulated by an awareness of the importance of nonverbal components of communication, as a result of various research findings. Birdwhistell (1970) for example, points out that the average person only speaks for a total of ten to eleven minutes daily, with the remainder of the communication time being taken up with nonverbal signals. Thus, it is obvious that the nonverbal channel is of vital import in social interaction.

Another indicator of the importance of this channel is the fact that most social meaning (attitudes, emotions, feelings) is conveyed nonverbally. Where a contradiction exists between the verbal and the nonverbal social messages, then the nonverbal aspects will usually be believed. If someone yawns, looks at their watch and says in a disinterested tone of voice 'That's very interesting', the listener will not believe the verbal message. In this sense, actions speak louder than words. However, because humans are the only animal to have developed a systematic language, we tend to concentrate on the verbal messages conveyed. As a result, we are taught from childhood to watch what we say, but are not really taught to watch our body language. The result is that we generally have much greater control over the verbal than the nonverbal channel.

Psychiatric Implications

Differences between socially skilled and socially unskilled individuals are readily evident in nonverbal communication patterns. It has been clearly shown that depressed and anxious patients can be identified purely by observing their nonverbal patterns of behaviour. Depressed patients are characterised by lack of eye contact, eyes looking down and away from the other person, downward angle of the head, down-turned mouth and absence of hand movements. As a result, depressed people are unrewarding and uninteresting to interact with, they are therefore avoided by others, and this in turn perpetuates their depressed state. Anxious patients manifest more self-stroking, twitching and tremors in hand movements, lower duration of eye contact, greater rigidity in posture and fewer smiles than the normal population. Again, these variations from the nonverbal norms cause interaction problems for anxious patients. Their continual movements of the hands, lack of smiles and shorter mutual gaze is off-putting for others, and does not enhance the possibility of relationship development with strangers.

Other psychiatric patients have also been found to have marked abnormalities in nonverbal communication. Autistic people are characterised by extreme gaze aversion. Since eye contact is necessary for communication, this is a pattern that such patients may well employ in order to ensure that they can maintain their 'isolation from others'. Violent offenders seem to prefer greater inter-personal distance than normals, use more hand gestures, and look more but smile less frequently. These patterns tend to result in the increased likelihood of being involved in aggressive incidents, since the violent offender is likely to become upset if someone is standing at a normal distance, and may misinterpret this as an aggressive approach. Coupled with their tendency to stare and not smile, this will be regarded by others as threatening behaviour. Finally, schizophrenics seem to look less when discussing personal matters, although they adopt normal gaze patterns when discussing neutral subject matter. Again, the abnormal eye contact pattern employed when discussing personal matters is likely to inhibit the development of inter-personal relationships where personal details will have to be discussed.

Most patients who experience difficulties in inter-personal encounters will have problems with nonverbal communication. Not only do many patients have problems with their own non-verbal behaviour, but they have also been found to be poorer than normals in decoding and interpreting nonverbal cues conveyed by others. They tend to misjudge these cues and overemphasise the speech content. As Bull (1983) points out:

> The consistent finding that psychiatric groups are inferior to normal groups in the decoding of non-verbal cues, and that they attribute less importance to such cues than normal groups would suggest that instruction in decoding may also be an appropriate form of therapy.

As a result, careful attention needs to be paid to this channel during SST.

The Nature of Nonverbal Communication

Nonverbal communication can be defined as all forms of human communication apart from the purely verbal message (the words used). Using this definition, the term nonverbal therefore encompasses the vocal dimension associated with the verbal message. In other words it includes the tone, pitch, volume, accent, speed etc. of the voice, an area of study referred to as *paralanguage* (how something is said as opposed to what is said). It also incorporates the area of body language which includes body contact, proximity, orientation, posture, body movements, gaze, facial expressions and appearance. We will be looking briefly at each of these elements later in the chapter.

These forms of nonverbal communication serve a number of purposes:

They can Totally Replace Speech.   This happens in many contexts, the prime example being sign language amongst the deaf and dumb where speech is not possible. Other special instances include traffic policemen, race-course bookies, and TV producers in the studio. In everyday interactions, nonverbal methods can also often replace speech. We can let others know we like or dislike them, agree or disagree with them, and pass other such messages by nonverbal means alone. Indeed, saying verbally to someone 'I dislike you' may lead to aggression, whereas conveying this message non-verbally and subtly (e.g. by orientating the body away from the person, looking less at them) will usually have a more acceptable result. Socially skilled individuals will have a greater capacity both for sending messages nonverbally, and for interpreting such messages from others.

They can Complement the Verbal Message. Nonverbal behaviours are generally used to give emphasis to the verbal message. Someone who says they are very angry will be expected to act angrily and, as mentioned earlier, if there is a contradiction then the nonverbal signals will be believed. Nonverbals can also facilitate the transmission of information, as when someone uses gestures to illustrate an explanation.

They are Used to Regulate and Control the Flow of Communication. When two people are interacting they use nonverbal signals to indicate when it is the other person's turn to speak. The person finishing speaking will raise or lower the final syllable, and look directly at the listener. By so doing the speaker is conveying the message 'I have now finished, it is your turn to speak'. Similarly, dominance in interaction is usually conveyed nonverbally, whereby the person who wants to control the interaction will speak more loudly, will choose a position of control (e.g. the top end of the table as with the board chairman), and will interrupt others.

They Provide Feedback. In social interaction people constantly monitor one another, in order to gauge reactions. When we are talking to someone we will periodically look at them to check if they are still listening, are interested, and so on. As discussed in Chapter 4 this feedback plays an important role in inter-personal communication, since it influences our future behaviour. Patients, therefore, need to learn to be as sensitive as possible to nonverbal forms of feedback and to improve their accuracy in interpreting this information.

They Help Define Relationships between People. A good example of this can be observed within a general hospital where uniforms are used to signal the role, function and status of the various professionals. Similarly, in church usually only one person will be dressed in a religious uniform and allowed access to the pulpit. A less formal example is a male walking with his arm round a female to signal to others 'she is mine' (although this sense of belonging can be formalised by means of engagement and wedding rings). This is an important function of nonverbal communication, since it facilitates the flow of communication and circumvents any role confusion. The more implicit aspects of this function need to be explored with patients. For example, at a selection interview it would not be acceptable for the interviewee to move his or her chair too far from its initial placing, without being given permission to do so by the interviewer, since to do so might well affect the relationship between the two.

They Provide Guidelines Regarding Appropriate Behaviour in Various Settings. At a very formal level this might include predetermined and ritualised verbal and nonverbal responses, as at a wedding ceremony in church, or a graduation ceremony at university. In most situations, however, certain behaviours will be regarded as appropriate or inappropriate. One does not lie on the floor during selection interviews, kiss strangers in the street, or sing loudly at the cinema! Yet, the manifestation of bizarre or inappropriate nonverbal communication is the hallmark of many patients. During SST, the importance of employing appropriate nonverbal behaviours should be emphasised, and situations which the patient is likely to encounter should be explored in relation to acceptable nonverbal responses.

These six functions encapsulate the main dimensions of nonverbal communication, and should be borne in mind in relation to the following sections on the component elements of nonverbal communications.

Body Contact

The use of touch is a very important, yet very sensitive, aspect of human interaction. In infancy, touch seems to be crucial for the psychological wellbeing of the child, and children who are deprived of touch at this stage of development seem to suffer adversely in later life, often finding difficulty in relating to others. However, while it is quite acceptable for young children to give and receive high levels of body contact, as the child grows the amount of touch in which he or she engages decreases. In many Western countries there are low levels of touch between adult individuals, although there are cultural differences here. In one particular study, Jourard (1966) compared levels of touching between opposite sex couples in cafés throughout the world. In a one-hour period he noted the following amount of touch in various locations: San Juan (Puerto Rico) 180; Paris 110; London 0. Thus, any study of body contact must take into account prevailing cultural norms.

The main categories of touch between adults include:

Social. During greetings and partings people often engage in some form of bodily contact. This may include a handshake, kiss on the cheek, kiss on the lips or a hug. The degree of touch will depend upon the relationship and its depth (e.g. old friend or slight acquaintance), as well as the prevailing circumstances. Thus at an airport departure or arrival lounge it is usually possible to estimate how long a person has been, or is going, away by the extent of touch they receive. Patients may need to learn when, how, and in what ways, to use body contact.

Affectionate. As a male-female relationship develops, so the levels of touch increase and become more intimate. However, any attempt to speed up this process will usually meet with a rebuttal and termination of the relationship. Thus, as mentioned in Chapter 1 the typical progression of touch in courtship is: hand to hand, arm to shoulder, arm to waist, mouth to mouth, hand to head, hand to body, mouth to breast, hand to genitals, genitals to genitals. Anyone who engages in touch (other than handshake) too early in a relationship may be greeted with suspicion.

Consoling. Where someone is deeply upset, touch can be used as a form of comfort or consolation. A good example of this occurs following bereavement when the bereaved will receive touch from others in the form of handshake, holding hands, arm round the shoulder or hugging.

Ritual. Many ceremonies include formalised touch, such as the handshake at prize-giving or the kiss following the wedding vows.

Occupation. In numerous professions touch is an integral part of the job, as with doctors, nurses, dentists and physiotherapists.

Aggressive. Touch can be used as an indication of aggressiveness, usually along a continuum including bumping into, pushing, slapping, punching and kicking.

Facilitating. This occurs when someone is helping another individual. It would include assisting an elderly or infirm person up a flight of stairs, or aiding a blind person in a strange environment.

Accidental. Interestingly, when two people touch accidentally, they usually apologise to one another. In many cases such touch is unavoidable, as at a crowded soccer match, and in these instances it will be accepted as an inevitable part of the situation.

Proximity

This refers to the inter-personal distance that people maintain when interacting with one another. Four main zones of proximity have been identified, namely:

1. Intimate: 0-18 inches. This is the distance at which people who have an intimate relationship may interact. It facilitates close bodily contact, and private discussions.
2. Personal: 18 inches-4 feet. Close friends will usually interact at this distance, and informal conversations are conducted within this zone.
3. Social/consultative: 4 feet-12 feet. This is the distance at which a professional will normally interact with a client. Solicitors, accountants, and bank managers will usually interact with their clients at this distance. The more impersonal the professional interaction the greater the distance will be between interactors.
4. Public: 12 feet +. Important persons, such as monarchs, prime ministers and presidents will normally retain this level of distance from others, as will lecturers.

Appropriate use of inter-personal distance from others is

important in social encounters. We do not like people who violate the cultural norms in either direction, by being 'too close for comfort' or 'very standoffish'. Initial conversations with strangers will usually take place at the outer edge of the personal zone. If either person does not want to pursue the interaction they will move out of this zone. As a relationship develops, the inter-personal distance will gradually be reduced. Thus, we stand closer to people we like. Other factors are also important: we come closer when standing than when sitting; status differences exist in that high status people can approach and come close to low status people but not vice versa; and finally, sex differences exist here in that two males will stand further apart than will two females or a male/female dyad. These points need to be considered when exploring this aspect of patient behaviour during SST.

Orientation

Orientation refers to the spatial positions that people take up in relation to one another. How we orientate our bodies in interaction will provide information for others. For example, if we do not like someone or do not want to interact with them, we will usually orientate our bodies away from them. This may involve crossing of the legs away from the person when seated, or turning slightly away from them towards someone else. Thus in Figure 7.1, B is gradually orientating himself away from C and saying nonverbally 'I'd rather talk to A than to you'.

Certain positions facilitate the control of an interaction. The

Figure 7.1: Orientation Example

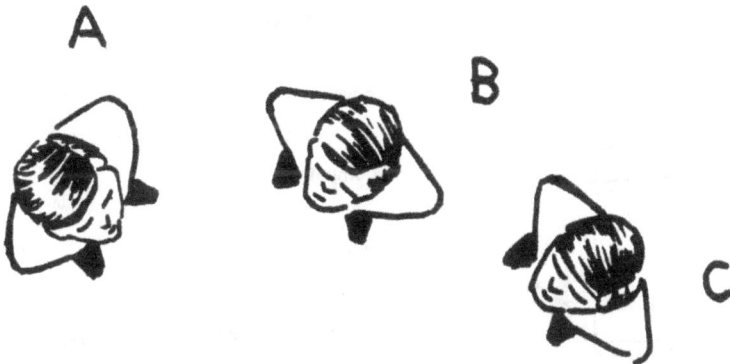

chairman of the board will sit at the top of the table to see every-one clearly and thereby ensure that he maintains his authority. Control is also conveyed by greater height, so the judge passes sentence from on high, the priest preaches from the pulpit and the teacher stands while pupils sit. This facet is linked with childhood when adults who have control of children are always taller than them. Hence we use expressions such as 'He is someone to be looked up to' 'She is over him at work' 'He is above her' to indi-cate superiority linked to position. Interestingly, small people who want to be dominant often tilt their heads back to give the appear-ance of looking down on others.

Choice of seating position is also important. As Figure 7.2 indicates different seating arrangements convey different messages, and this is an important element of communication. In public places it is necessary to be aware of the orientation norms. For example, position No. 4 in Figure 7.2 would usually be adopted if there was only one table with dining space in a restaurant and one person was already sitting at it. Similarly if we are sitting in a nearly empty pub or library, we will be unhappy if someone sits beside us without giving some explanation or justification.

These are some of the elements of orientation that are of rele-vance during inter-personal interaction. Patients need to be aware both of the significance of choosing certain types of orientation, and of the meaning being conveyed by others through their choice of orientation.

Figure 7.2: Seating Orientations

Seating Position	Usual Meaning
1.	Having a discussion
2.	Competing
3.	Working together
4.	Independent action

Posture

As mentioned earlier, certain types of psychiatric patients can be identified from the posture they adopt. Anxious patients often portray a stiff, rigid posture, while depressed patients display a slouched, drooping posture. For these patients, a knowledge of the meaning and effects of posture is very important.

There are three main categories of posture:

(1) Standing
(2) Sitting, squatting or kneeling
(3) Lying

In social encounters standing and sitting postures are important. Posture is used to make judgements regarding attitudes and emotions. We take posture into consideration when making decisions about whether people are interested in what we are saying (forward lean when seated; upright posture with head tilted) or are totally disinterested (slouched in chair, drooping head). We also make interpretations about whether people like us or not based partially upon posture. A closed posture with arms and legs tightly crossed usually signals that the person does not want to interact freely, whereas a more open posture with hands and/or legs uncrossed is taken as a sign of friendship. Estimates of depression, excitement, happiness, confidence and many other emotions, are guided by the postures people adopt.

For these reasons, posture is an important dimension of communication. Failure to adopt the appropriate posture can adversely influence the outcome of an interaction. At a selection interview, where interest and attentiveness are expected from interviewees, a depressed or disinterested posture will result in non-selection, as will continual posture shifts. Furthermore, someone who continually displays these types of posture will find difficulty in many social situations. Interestingly when two people like one another they will adopt similar or even identical postures during interaction, a process known as 'posture-mirroring'. This process should be explored and practised during SST.

Body Movements

This area encompasses movements in the three main areas of the body described below.

(1) Hands and arms. Movements here, commonly referred to as gestures, can be either communicative or self-orientated. Communicative gestures are often, although not always, linked with speech and help facilitate the verbal message being conveyed. There are many examples of communicative gestures including the following:

Movement	Message
Thumbs-up	Success
Banging fist on table	Anger
Waving hand with palm outwards	Goodbye
Wagging index finger	Come here
Arms stiff and outstretched with palms outwards	Stop or stay away

These signals are readily recognisable with or without speech. In addition, we use gestures to emphasise what is being said. For example saying 'these are three main points' while raising three fingers, or saying 'it is oval shaped' while making an oval shape with the hands. These communicative gestures help to convey interest and promote understanding.

Self-orientated gestures, on the other hand, can be very distracting and can detract from the verbal message. Such gestures include wringing the hands, stroking or scratching oneself, twisting a ring, and nail biting. They are indicative of the emotional state of the person and usually serve as forms of tension release. People who indulge in repeated self-orientated gestures are regarded as being anxious or neurotic, and difficult to communicate with. On the other hand, a complete absence of hand or arm movements is also inappropriate in social interaction, being characteristic of depression. Thus, a balance of such movements should be encouraged during SST, with patients learning about the disadvantages of using too many self-orientated gestures or too few communicative gestures.

(2) Head and shoulders. Head nods can be either slow and deliberate indicating 'I am listening; continue talking', or very fast to signal 'I know what you are telling me; get on with it'. Similarly, shaking the head slowly can mean 'I disagree', shaking it very quickly usually indicates 'I strongly disagree'. The intensity of head movements will, therefore, change their

meaning. There are various meanings associated with head movements including:

Head Movement	Message
Cocked to one side	Puzzlement
Head down, thumb on one side of forehead fingers on other side	Thinking
Tossed in the air	Defiance
Tilted back	Dominance
Head bowed, hands covering face	Despair
Head bowed	Sadness

Movements of the shoulders are limited in terms of social interaction, although we shrug our shoulders to indicate that we do not know what is being asked, or stiffen our shoulders to convey tension.

(3) Legs and feet. This area of the body is not often explicitly used during inter-personal communication. One possible exception is where two people play 'footsie' under the table! Apart from this, implicit meanings are often conveyed through leg and foot movements. Continual crossing and uncrossing of the legs or shuffling of the feet are viewed as signs of tension, similar to self-orientated gestures. Together, these are referred to as 'social leakages', wherein the person is socially leaking to others the fact that he or she is nervous or anxious. Such leakages are taken either as signs of lack of self-control, or as indicators that the person is being deceitful, and give a negative impression to others. Thus, at selection interviews someone who displays a large number of these leakages will be unlikely to be selected. Another implicit meaning associated with the legs occurs when someone who sits with legs crossed away from another person is viewed as not wanting to communicate with that person. In addition, as mentioned when discussing posture, someone who sits with arms and legs tightly crossed is viewed as not wanting to participate.

These are some of the meanings associated with body movements. In fact there are innumerable variations of movement with different meanings, and patients should be sensitised to this area in general so that they become more aware of the effects of such movements.

Facial Expressions

Judgements about the emotional state of another person seem to rely heavily upon the interpretation of facial expressions. In particular, movements of the eyebrows and mouth are used to signal different types of emotion. Slight variations of movements in either or both of these regions will result in changed interpretations of emotional state. Some examples of this are presented diagrammatically in Figure 7.3, in terms of the extremes of movement of eyebrows and mouth. In between these extremes, however, lies a whole plethora of different types of facial expression. Ekman and Friesen (1982) have identified a total of 46 *separate* facial movements (single action units) such as 'inner brow raiser', 'lip corner depressor', 'cheek puffer', 'nostril dilator' and 'wink'. It is obvious that the variety of combinations of two or more of these movements will result in an enormous total number of facial expressions.

It also seems likely that many of these variations will be taken as

Figure 7.3: Effects of Eyebrow and Mouth Variations on Facial Expressions

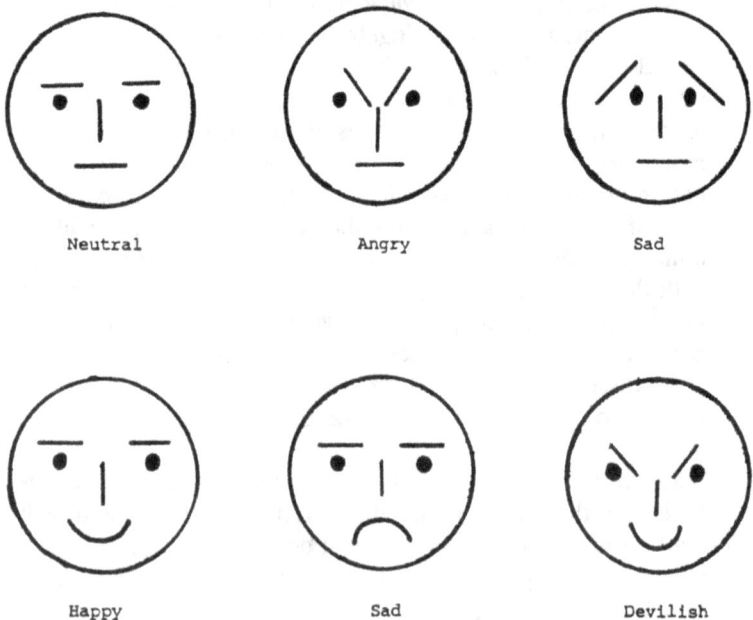

Neutral   Angry   Sad

Happy   Sad   Devilish

having a similar meaning. This is underlined by the fact that a number of studies have reported seven main groups of facial expression which are representative of the following emotions:

(1) Happiness
(2) Sadness
(3) Fear
(4) Interest
(5) Anger
(6) Surprise
(7) Disgust/contempt

As well as the eyebrows and mouth, other movements include movements of the nostrils, nose and tongue. Thus, when we are angry we may flare our nostrils, when we disapprove we turn up our noses, and if we want to be cheeky or provocative we may display our tongues. Again, these elements are concerned primarily with the communication of emotion. Facial expression can also communicate attitudes, as when we roll our eyes at person A while person B is speaking, to indicate 'What a bore B is!'.

Many psychiatric patients are characterised by lack of variation of facial expressions. Depressives and anxious patients smile very infrequently and are therefore unrewarding to interact with. Violent offenders also tend to smile very little, and this is a behavioural style which probably results in them being viewed by others as aggressive (when taken in conjunction with other behaviours they display as discussed earlier). It is therefore important to focus upon the dimension of facial expressions during SST, and to sensitise patients to the importance of improving this aspect of their social presentation.

Gaze

The use of different patterns of gaze serves a number of important functions during social interaction. Direct mutual gaze or eye-to-eye contact is usually a prerequisite to beginning an interaction. In order to obtain service in a bar or restaurant it is necessary to 'catch the eye' of the waiter. Similarly, males and females signal interest in one another by 'making eyes' or looking directly to indicate that interaction is desired. Thus, initial eye contact communicates a desire or willingness to participate with another person. Equally, avoidance of eye contact at this stage is usually taken as an indicator of disinterest, or lack of desire to get involved with another person.

The facial expressions that accompany eye contact and indeed all other nonverbal and verbal behaviours, as well as situational factors, need to be taken into account when evaluating eye contact patterns. For example, a courting couple may stare lovingly at one another for long periods of time. However, if one male stares coldly at another male, this can be taken as an aggressive or threatening display. Indeed, dominant people will stare more frequently than affiliative people during inter-personal encounters, and will also look directly at the other person both when speaking and when listening. On average, in Western society, the listener will look at the speaker twice as much as the speaker will look at the listener. Thus, person A who is speaking will look away for much of the time, but will also look periodically at person B for feedback as to how the message is being received. B, on the other hand, will tend to look frequently at A to convey interest in, and attention to, what is being said. Dominant and aggressive people, however, will deviate from this pattern by staring at the listener when they are speaking.

Gaze also controls turn-taking during communication. When the speaker is reaching the end of his utterance, they will look directly at the listener and pause, to signal that they have finished speaking and it is the other's turn. Such signals obviously facilitate the flow of interaction. Another function of gaze is to indicate liking for another, since we look more at people we like or find attractive and less at those we dislike. We also look less when embarrassed or feeling guilty. If a group of people are interacting and there is a sudden lull in the conversation, during which no-one can think of anything to say, eye contact will be avoided until someone breaks the silence thereby overcoming the embarrassment. Likewise, if we feel guilty or have something to hide, we tend to engage in less eye contact. This can be observed at an early age in young children who have committed a misdemeanour, and will then avert their gaze when confronted. In adult life, psychiatrists may put patients on a couch and sit in a chair behind them, to overcome any added embarrassment that direct eye contact may cause when discussing difficult personal problems. In everyday conversations, we are often suspicious of people who do not look at us since we interpret this as a sign that they have something to conceal.

There are, however, cultural and sex differences in eye contact patterns. It has been found that Arabs and Greeks look more during social interaction than Americans or Europeans. However, it has also been found that some groups of black American males have a gaze pattern of looking more while speaking and less while listening, which is the converse of the pattern for whites. These differences in gaze patterns probably result in difficulties in interaction between the black and white males, with the whites regarding blacks as aggressive because they look while speaking. More research is needed into subcultural variations in gaze to ascertain whether any similar differences exist among other groups. Differences have also been found between the sexes, in that females look more both at males and other females, while males look more at females than they do at other males.

Abnormal gaze patterns are symptomatic of many psychiatric patients. Depressed, anxious, schizophrenic and autistic patients all demonstrate a lower duration of eye contact than normals. Most patients who are diagnosed as socially inadequate will demonstrate some degree of abnormality in eye contact, either looking too little or too much. Thus, an analysis of this element is important during SST.

Appearance

It is possible to control some aspects of appearances more easily than others. Clothes, and hair colour and style, can be manipulated fairly easily, and, although more difficult, so can weight and overall body shape. Other aspects can be changed by means of surgery, such as shape of nose, removal of wrinkles and so on. Finally, there are aspects, including height, that can be manipulated only slightly, if at all.

Appearance serves a number of functions. It is an indicator of self-image, so that someone who is smartly dressed and well groomed is deemed to have a good self-image, and is regarded as being confident and in control of their situation. Conversely, someone who is unkempt and shabbily dressed is viewed as having a low self-image and seen as lacking in confidence and control. It is often possible to recognise psychiatric patients purely on the basis of appearance, because they will frequently take little care with this aspect of self-presentation. Ill-fitting or mismatched clothing and dishevelled hair are symptomatic of certain patients. Thus, depressed patients, may make little effort to present themselves in a good light saying that they 'see little point'.

Yet attractiveness is an important facet of inter-personal communication, since attractive people receive more attention from
others. Attractiveness is more than physical features, and factors
that have been found to be important in ratings of attractiveness
include cleanliness and dress. It is therefore important to
encourage patients to maximise the potential benefits to be
obtained from their appearance. Patients should be made aware of
the importance of appearance in many contexts. For example, it is
associated with certain job roles, as in the uniforms worn by many
professions including policemen, firemen and nurses. It is also
utilised to indicate identification with a particular group, such as
businessmen, hell's angels, punk rockers or hippies. Finally, it is
employed to convey interest in others as when we dress up to go
on a date or to a selection interview.

Paralanguage

This refers to *how* something is said as opposed to *what* is said.
The actual meaning of an utterance is greatly influenced by the
way in which it is delivered. Changes in tone, pitch, volume and
speed can affect the message being conveyed. Consider the following example of how a change in emphasis can effect the meaning
of a statement:

(1)   JOHN invited me to his flat
(1a) John is the person who invited me; no-one else
(2)   John INVITED me to his flat
(2a) John issued an invitation; I did not go uninvited
(3)   John invited ME to his flat
(3a) John invited me, not you or anyone else
(4)   John invited me to HIS flat
(4a) This is why we went to John's flat, and not to anyone else's
(5)   John invited me to his FLAT
(5a) This is why I went to his flat and not to some other place.

People who can effect variations in their speech style are, not
surprisingly, regarded as more interesting and stimulating than
those who speak in a dull, flat monotone. Good teachers, politicians and raconteurs are aware of the importance of changes in
vocal pattern for maintaining attention. However, individuals who
have problems in social interaction will often have problems in

relation to speech style. At an extreme level this can take the shape of severe speech dysfluencies, in the form of stuttering or stammering, where the intervention of a speech therapist may be appropriate. At a less extreme level, it may be a matter of encouraging patients to inject more enthusiasm into their utterances, although it must be realised that even small changes in this area can be difficult to achieve. Other aspects of paralanguage that can be studied include the use of pauses, and refraining from interruptions during social interaction.

Self-disclosure

A great deal of social interaction is concerned with participants giving opinions, relating feelings and making statements about a wide variety of topics; in other words making disclosures. Such disclosures can be about objective matters ('It is six o'clock') or they can involve a subjective dimension regarding the speaker ('I am tired'). This latter type of disclosure is referred to as self-disclosure, which can be defined as the process whereby one individual verbally and/or nonverbally shares with another some item of personal information.

Self-disclosure, therefore, involves both verbal and nonverbal communication since both channels will convey information of a personal nature. Verbal self-disclosures are statements in which the individual reveals personal information about himself. Nonverbal self-disclosures are behaviours displayed by an individual that convey to others an impression of his or her attitudes or feelings. As discussed earlier, facial expressions, posture, gaze, paralanguage and all the other features of nonverbal communication are the means whereby we provide information about our emotional state. Thus we can 'say' nonverbally 'I am very happy' by smiling, having an unright posture and looking at the other person. An important difference between verbal and nonverbal self-disclosure is that we tend to have much greater control over the former than the latter. Unfortunately, many patients will demonstrate problems with both forms of self-disclosure. It is necessary, therefore, for the nurse to have an understanding of this skill and of its effects in inter-personal encounters, in order to encourage patients to improve their use of self-disclosure during SST.

Features of Self-disclosure

The four main features of self-disclosure are as follows:

(1) The use of the personal pronoun 'I' or some other personal self-reference pronoun such as 'my' or 'mine'. While these words may be implied from the context of the speaker's utterances, their presence serves to remove any ambiguity about whether or not the statement being made is a self-disclosure. For this reason, the basic reference point for all self-disclosures should be a personal pronoun. Compare, for example the statements:

A. Selection interviews can create a great amount of stress
B. I find selection interviews very stressful.

In A it is not immediately clear whether the speaker is making a general statement, or referring to his own feelings about attending selection interviews. The use of the personal pronoun 'I' in B, however, serves to clarify the nature of the statement as a self-disclosure.

(2) Self-disclosures can be about either facts or feelings. When two people meet for the first time, it is more likely that they will focus upon factual disclosures (name, occupation, place of residence) while keeping any feeling disclosures at a fairly superficial level ('I hate crowded parties', 'I like rock music'). This is largely because the expression of personal feeling involves more risk and places the discloser in a more vulnerable position. At the same time, however, deep levels of disclosure may be made to a complete stranger providing that we feel sure we will never meet the person again. Thus two strangers sitting beside one another on a long-haul plane journey who discover that their encounter is likely to be 'one-off' may reveal personal information and feelings, which would not do if they were planning to meet one another on a regular basis.

Generally speaking, the expression of deep feeling or of high levels of factual disclosure (e.g. 'I was in prison for 5 years') will increase as a relationship develops. Indeed, some patients will find difficulty in developing inter-personal relationships by over-disclosing too early, often during a first encounter. Factual and feeling disclosures at a deeper level can be regarded as a sign of commitment to a relationship. Two people who are in love will usually expect to give and receive disclosures about their feelings — especially towards one another. They will also want to know everything about one another. In such a relationship there will be a high level of trust, just as there will be in the confession box, a doctor's surgery or a counselling session (areas where disclosures will also be high).

(3) Self-disclosures can be about one's own personal experience or they can be about one's personal reaction to the feelings being expressed by someone else. Consider the following:

Ann   I haven't been sleeping too well lately. I work until midnight every night, and yet nothing seems to sink in. I'm really worried about these exams. What will I do if I fail them?

Bob   You know, I'm very concerned about you. It seems to me that you are working too much and not getting enough sleep.

Cecil Yes. I remember when I was sitting my final exams. I was worried about them too. The doctor gave me sleeping tablets but I didn't want to take them because ...

Here, Bob's response focuses upon Ann and the feeling she had initially expressed, whereas Cecil's response is more of a 'me, too' reaction. If Cecil continually responds in this manner the result will be that other people will tend to avoid him, and he will be regarded as a self-centred, conversational bore.

(4) Self-disclosure can be about the past ('I was born in Belfast: as a child I hated my father'), the present ('I am married: I am very pleased'), or the future ('I hope to get promotion: when I retire I will go back to Ireland'). One situation in which people are expected to self-disclose in terms of facts and feelings about the past, present and future, is in the selection interview. Candidates will be asked to talk about their previous experience or education, to say why they have applied for the job and to outline their aspirations. The depth of self-disclosure required will vary from one interview to another, and at an executive level the candidate may be asked to answer the question 'What type of person are you?'.

Other Aspects of Self-disclosure

In addition to the above central features of self-disclosure, a number of other important aspects should be borne in mind.

The Amount of Information Provided. As Figure 7.4 indicates, self-disclosures can be assessed along two dimensions, namely breadth and depth. Thus, the breadth (or total number) of self-disclosures can be narrow or broad, while the depth can be shallow or deep. It is possible to disclose a lot about oneself (broad) at a shallow level. On the other hand, deep self-disclosures tend to be less frequent in social interaction. Derlega and Chaikin (1975) give an example of a questionnaire designed to measure both breadth and depth of disclosures. Examples of shallow levels of disclosure given in this questionnaire include 'Laws that I would like to see put into effect', 'Whether I would rather live in an apartment or a house after getting married'; and deeper levels such as 'How frequently I like to engage in sexual activity', 'The kinds of things I do that I don't want people to watch'. As mentioned earlier, deeper disclosures are more appropriate once relationships have been built up.

Figure 7.4: Dimensions of Self-disclosure

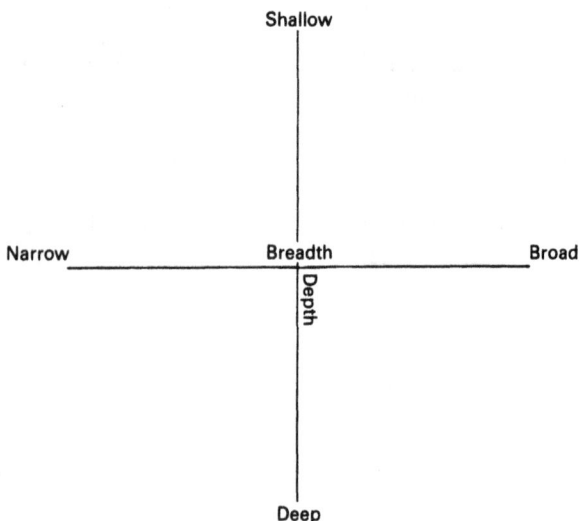

The Ease with which the Person Discloses Information. Some individuals will be more reluctant, for whatever reason, to talk about themselves. This may be due to personality (introverts will talk less generally, and will tend to self-disclose less than extroverts), upbringing (parents may have taught the child to be more closed than open) or lack of learning about how and what to disclose in social interaction.

The Outcome of the Disclosure for both Discloser and Listener. The outcome may be positive or negative for either or both. Some individuals disclose negative information about themselves too often. ('I am depressed', 'I have piles'). Equally, some individuals make negative disclosures about the listener ('You have a lot of spots', 'I see you have a problem with dandruff'). In both instances, this type of person will have difficulties in interpersonal relationships, since the outcome of their disclosures is negative and unrewarding for the listener. Such people need to learn to be more positive and rewarding in the information which they disclose.

Self-disclosures can be True or False. In some instances an individual may disclose false information in order to impress. This type of disclosure can place the person under a lot of stress. In effect, the greater the discrepancy between the real self and the image of the self as portrayed to others, the greater will be the pressures and tensions within the individual, since the person has constantly to maintain the facade that has been presented. In extreme cases this can lead to breakdown. One example of this is where someone gives the impression of being confident and in control, when under the surface they are full of self-doubt and uncertainty, and yet feel unable to admit this since they feel that if they do their image will be irrevocably damaged. Eventually such a mismatch can no longer be maintained, and the person ends up being unable to cope.

Appropriateness. This is perhaps the most crucial aspect of self-disclosure. Each disclosure needs to be evaluated in the light of the context in which it occurs. There is research evidence to suggest that neurotics do not take this factor into account, and are inflexible in that their pattern of disclosures does not vary between situations. While there are no hard and fast rules about the exact appropriateness of self-disclosure in every situation, there are some general indicators. Self-disclosures are more appropriate:

(1) From low status to high status individuals but not vice versa. Thus, workers may disclose personal problems to their supervisors, but the reverse does not usually happen. This is because for a supervisor to disclose personal information to a subordinate would cause a loss of face which would affect the status relationship.

(2) When the listener is not flooded with them. As Figure 7.5 illustrates, there is a relationship between psychological adjustment and self-disclosure in that individuals who are extremely high or low disclosers will have low adjustment.

(3) Depending upon the roles of the interactors. For example, we may disclose information to our spouses which we would not disclose to our children.

(4) Depending upon the setting. Thus, we do not normally discuss bowel problems during meal-times!

(5) At deeper levels later in a relationship. Exceptions to this include interacting with a stranger who will never be seen again, or in a crisis situation (e.g. counselling, the confessional).

Figure 7.5: Relationship between Adjustment and Disclosure

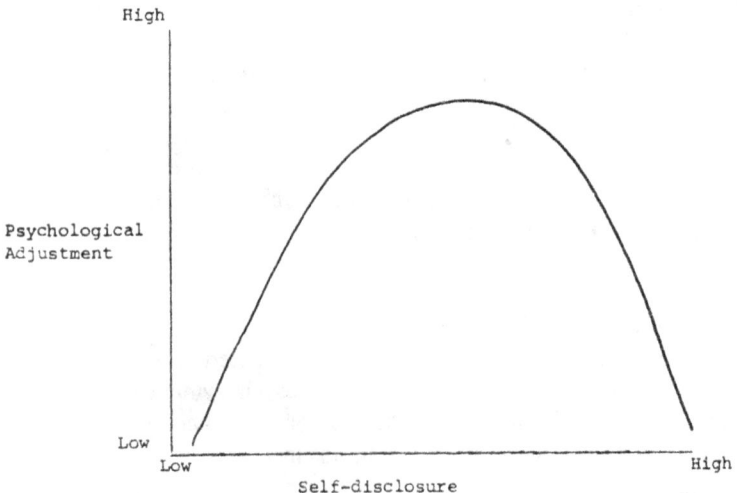

The Effectiveness of the Disclosure is also Important.   Does the disclosure help the individual to obtain his or her goals? If an individual's disclosures are ineffective in so doing, then it is necessary to examine the nature and pattern of such disclosures. This is important during the assessment phase of SST. The nurse will need to ascertain the typical self-disclosure style of the patient across situations, and the effects of such disclosures.

Functions of Self-disclosure

The skill of self-disclosure serves a number of purposes in social interaction. It is often used to *open conversations* especially with strangers. The following is a typical example of many initial encounters:

Robert	Hello, my name is Robert. What's yours?
Dervilla	Dervilla.
Robert	Dervilla. That's an unusual name. Are you from here?
Dervilla	No. I was born in Scotland but I've lived here for six years.
Robert	That's interesting. Actually I'm from New Zealand originally, but my parents came to live here when I was four. What's your surname?
Dervilla	Kane. What's yours?
Robert	Dixon, with an X. I work just down the road in the family business. You may have seen it, the timber yard on Main Street.

In this setting both parties are giving and receiving personal information about one another, in order to build up a picture of the other person. This enables a decision to be made about whether the relationship is worth pursuing. It is therefore important that *reciprocation* of disclosures occurs at this stage. If one person discloses nothing or over-discloses, this will upset the expected balance, and may well persuade the other person to terminate the encounter.

Reciprocation is also important in that many people have a fear of disclosing too much about their thoughts and feelings, since they feel that they may not be understood or will be subjected to ridicule. Indeed in many subcultures self-disclosure will be actively discouraged with the child being told to 'keep himself to himself' or 'tell people what they need to know'. This attitude then persists into later life where respect is often given to the person who 'plays his cards close to his chest'. While in a game of poker it is wise not to disclose too much, either verbally or nonverbally, the attitude of avoiding self-disclosure can cause problems for people. It can become a burden not being able to tell others about personal matters, and having to keep things bottled up. Self-disclosure can have a therapeutic effect, by enabling us to 'get it off our chest', which is why counselling, the confessional or discussing something with a close friend can make us feel better. Indeed, it is interesting to note that, when people may not be able to utilise one of these channels, they often use substitutes such as keeping a personal diary, talking to a pet, or conversing with God. However, the initial dangers of self-disclosure are such that we expect an equal commitment to this process from people with whom we may wish to develop a relationship. For this reason, reciprocation is expected in the early stages of interaction. In relation to the poker analogy it is a case of the individual wanting to see all the cards on the table!

Where reciprocation of self-disclosures does not occur, three types of situations will usually prevail:

(1) The person making the disclosures is not really interested in the listener. This type of person's need is so great that he or she wants to tell all, without worrying about the effect this may have upon the listener. The speaker is simply using the listener as a receptacle into which he pours his disclosures. This is quite common when someone is undergoing some form of inner turmoil, and needs a friendly ear to encourage the ventilation of fears and emotions. To use another analogy, the listener becomes a 'wailing wall' for the speaker. In certain circumstances this is acceptable, as in counselling and therapy. In other instances, however, it can cause problems. There is evidence that neurotics send many more self-disclosures than they receive, with resulting problems in social interaction.

(2) The person who is receiving the disclosures does not care about the speaker. In this case the speaker is foolish to continue disclosing, since it is possible that the listener may use the disclosures against the speaker, either at the time of the disclosure or later.

(3) Neither one cares about the disclosures of the other. In this case there is no real relationship. If one person discloses, it is a monologue; if both disclose it is a dialogue in which exchanges

are superficial. A great deal of everyday, fleeting conversation falls into the latter category.

Relationship building can also be facilitated by two other functions of self-disclosure. Appropriate reciprocation of self-disclosure is a potent form of listening. In the transcript above, it is obvious that Robert and Dervilla are listening closely to one another, since their disclosures are closely linked and questions follow on from these disclosures. In this way, initial interest is conveyed in each other. Furthermore, by self-disclosing, both people can search for shared experiences (in the previous example, the fact that neither was born in the area where the interaction is taking place). This is normal during first encounters, where both parties search for common ground on which to build a conversation (this is discussed further later in this chapter).

Self-disclosure can also be used to heighten personal knowledge. This is exemplified by the saying 'How do I know what I think until I hear what I say?' The value of the 'talking cure' in therapy is a good example of how the process of allowing someone to freely express their thoughts, ideas, fears, problems etc. actually facilitates the individual's awareness of the type of person they are. It can also help people to understand their feelings and the reasons for them, in other words it encourages them to know themselves more fully. People who do not have access to a good listener may not only be denied the opportunity to heighten their self-awareness, they are also denied valuable feedback as to the validity and acceptability of their inner thoughts and feelings. By discussing such inner thoughts and feelings with others, we receive feedback as to whether these are experiences which others have as well, or whether they may be less common. As a result, we learn what it is acceptable and unacceptable to disclose.

These functions of self-disclosure can be illustrated with reference to the Johari Window developed by two psychologists, Joseph Luft and Harry Ingram (Luft, 1969). As depicted in Figure 7.6, this indicates four dimensions of the self. There are aspects known both by the self and by others (A): aspects unknown by the self but known to others (B) including personal mannerisms, annoying habits and so on; aspects known by the self but not revealed to others (C) such as embarrassing personal details, thoughts or feelings; and aspects unknown both to the self and others (D). By self-disclosing we increase the size of A and reduce

Figure 7.6: The Johari Window

	Known to Self	Unknown to Self
Known to Others	A	B
Unknown to Others	C	D

the size of the segments B, C and D. In other words, not only do we learn more about ourselves, but we also allow others to find out more about us, and thereby perhaps understand us more fully.

Improving Self-disclosure

From this analysis of self-disclosure, it will be clear that this is an important skill for many patients to develop. As Cozby (1973) states in a review of research:

> Persons with positive mental health ... are characterised by high disclosure to a few significant others and medium disclosure to others in the social environment. Individuals who are poorly adjusted ... are characterized by either high or low disclosure to virtually everyone.

Such an abnormal pattern of disclosure obviously affects the interpersonal functioning of the individual. Similarly, attention needs to be paid to nonverbal disclosures in these patients. Verbal and nonverbal disclosures need to be synchronised, in that if someone says 'I am very happy' they need to act happy.

In encouraging the improved usage of this skill the nurse should consider the following:

(1) The total number of disclosures made
(2) The depth of these disclosures
(3) The content of disclosures in different settings
(4) The nonverbal as well as verbal component
(5) The rewardingness of disclosures
(6) The reciprocal nature of disclosures.

Greetings and Partings

The beginnings and endings of social encounters have long been recognised as crucial phases in the establishment, development and maintenance of relationships (e.g. Roth, 1889). Lack of skill during an initial meeting with another person can result in an early termination by them of the interaction episode, just as lack of skill in closing an encounter can result in the complete termination of a relationship. Thus it is important for patients to know both how to get in to and get out of a conversation. These are two stages of inter-personal interaction which many patients find difficult, and which are, therefore, important areas of study during SST.

Although we will look at both of these stages separately, it should be noted that they are complementary, in that greeting behaviours are used to signal that an interaction is about to begin, while parting behaviours are used to signal the end of interaction. These complementary functions are underlined when we examine the behaviours associated with the three main phases involved in both greetings and partings between friends:

(A) Distant phase. When the individuals are at a distance, but within sight, the behaviours displayed include hand waving, eyebrow flashing (raising both eyebrows), smiling, head tossing and direct eye contact.
(B) Medium phase. At a closer interim distance but not within touching range, the individuals will avoid eye contact, smile and engage in a range of self-touching behaviours.
(C) Close phase. At this phase the individuals will engage in direct eye contact, and bodily contact (shake hands, hug or kiss), will smile and make appropriate verbalisations.

In greetings, the sequence is ABC, while in partings it is the reverse sequence of CBA. At the greeting stage, these behaviours serve to underline the increased availability of the participants for inter-action, whereas at the parting stage they emphasise the fact that communication is gradually coming to an end.

While these three phases are typical of many greeting and parting episodes, a number of factors will influence the manner in which these episodes are enacted.

Acquaintance of the People Involved.   Different responses will be used with strangers as opposed to friends. The greeting stage will be more relaxed with friends who may use this stage just as a brief signalling point for beginning where they have recently left off, by using appropriate nonverbals coupled with a verbalisation such as 'Hi. How was the movie?' With strangers, greetings are usually much more formal, with the people involved having to find out about one another and search for common ground. Thus, there is often a process of 'feeling out' one another during first encounters, and interaction may not flow smoothly, since the individuals will not have developed a pattern of communication. Decisions will have to be made about whether interaction with the other is going to be worthwhile and rewarding, or tedious and unrewarding. Tacit agreements have to be worked out about who will be dominant and do most of the talking and who will be submissive and do more listening if a relationship is to be developed. Many of these decisions will be made during the first few minutes of interaction. Similarly, when parting, friends may exchange a casual 'Be seeing you' whereas strangers usually have to make a definite commit-ment to meet again, and make arrangements about when and where this will take place.

Duration of Separation.   People who have been, or are going, away for a long time will engage in more intensive and extensive behaviours than those involved in departures of a brief duration. This can be observed at any airport or large train station. Fairly accurate decisions can be made about the duration of departure based upon the ritualised behaviours displayed. There is much more eye contact, body contact and intense verbalisation involved in longer periods of separation. At the same time, however, some form of greeting and parting rituals are expected, regardless of the length of separation. Someone going home from work may just say to colleagues 'I'm away. See you in the morning', or on arrival say 'Good morning', and, although brief, these are acceptable and appropriate. In fact, we notice the absence of these rituals more than their presence ('what's wrong with John this morning? He walked past me without speaking').

Function of the Interaction.   Different forms of greeting and parting will be in evidence at a party, a counselling encounter and a selection interview. The degree of formality involved will increase across these three contexts, and this will be reflected in the greetings and partings. At a party, the function of greetings is usually to highlight the informal, friendly nature of the forthcoming event with the emphasis upon enjoyment, and the parting behaviours will reinforce that this has indeed occurred. At a counselling session where the function is to offer support, the greeting will be relaxed, yet caring and professional, as will the parting. Selection interviews on the other hand, are much more formal, involving candidates being assessed as to their suitability for a particular job, and this will be reflected in the formality of the opening and closing stages of the interview. Thus, the function of the interaction will have a direct bearing upon the nature of the greeting and parting behaviours employed.

Location of the Interaction.   As discussed in Chapter 4, a number of situational rules and norms set parameters for acceptable and unacceptable behaviour within any given context. Thus, different greetings and partings will be used in church as opposed to in a bar. Similarly, we use different openings and closings in our own home compared to when we are guests in someone else's home. It is therefore important for patients to be aware of the relevance of both the function and location of the interaction to the way in which greetings and partings are conducted.

Sex of Participants.   Differences in the behaviours associated with 'hellos' and 'goodbyes' have been noted between the sexes. When two adult males meet in our society, the main form of body contact is the handshake. When a female meets either another female or a male there tends to be a greater degree of body contact, in the form of a hug and/or kiss. It has also been noted, however that increasingly in the occupational context, females are adopting the male pattern of handshake only. Another difference is in the amount of eye contact, with two males looking less at one another than either two females, or a male and a female.

These factors all need to be borne in mind when considering what constitutes appropriate greetings and partings.

Greeting

The ritualised behaviour sequences associated with greetings serve a number of important functions in social interaction. The main functions are:

To Communicate the Desire for Interaction with the Other Person.   By smiling, nodding, looking at the other person and uttering a verbal greeting ('Hello. How are you?'), the friendly nature of the approach is underlined. This is very important, since it ensures that the approach is not viewed as aggressive. It is also a clear signal to the other that interaction is desired and a response expected. If this response is also friendly, then mutual agreement is being implicitly expressed for continuing with the interaction. If the initial greeting response is not reciprocated by the other, then this is a clear signal that no further communication is desired.

To Create a Good Impression on the Other Person and Increase their Desire to become Involved in Interaction.   This function is obviously closely linked to the first one. With strangers, a special effort should be made to appear as the type of person with whom they will find it rewarding to communicate. This is the reason why people dress up when going to a dance or a party, and why they make a special effort to appear happy and interested in someone they have just met. All of these factors serve to increase the attractiveness of the individual to others.

To Obtain an Appropriate Spatial Arrangement for Communication.   The greeting period allows people an opportunity to orient themselves in such a way as to facilitate communication. This would include choosing a suitable inter-personal distance from the other person, so that with strangers we will stand at a further distance than with friends. It will also involve not standing or sitting, while the other person remains seated or standing respectively. When meeting someone for the first time, it is important not to appear too familiar, while at the same time indicating a willingness to open up a conversation. Thus, the spatial factors should respect the privacy of the other, while enhancing the possibility of communication.

To Indicate the Degree of Formality Expected from the Inter-action. At a formal level, greetings usually include a brief firm handshake, eye contact, brief smile and a formal verbalisation ('How do you do': 'Pleased to meet you'). This type of greeting is prevalent in many business settings, where it is used to open up some form of negotiation. A much less formal greeting will take place between two teenage friends, where a smile, eyebrow flash, eye contact and brief verbalisation ('Hi') will be appropriate. These greetings serve to set the scene for the ensuing encounter, and lay down implicit guidelines about appropriate behaviour.

To Convey Commitment to an Ongoing Relationship. The degree of warmth demonstrated when greeting friends is often a good measure of the extent of our commitment to the friendship. Thus, if we have been friendly with someone, but decide that we would rather not continue to be so friendly with them in the future, this will be reflected in our greetings. Equally, if someone who normally greets us warmly, begins to reduce the warmth of their greetings we will take this as a sign either that something is wrong with them, or that they no longer wish to be so friendly with us.

To Communicate the Status Relationship between Interactors. In many settings, greetings are determined by status factors. A good example of this is the greeting between a monarch and others, where males are expected to bow and females to curtsy as signs of respect for the status of the monarch. Similarly, at selection inter-views, the interviewer (high status) will expect to take the lead and will not be happy with a candidate (lower status) who enters the room, comes round the desk, shakes hands, and proceeds to engage in small talk!

The first three of these functions are particularly important when starting interactions with strangers, an activity which many patients will find very difficult. Trower et al (1978) have identified three types of situations where strangers may meet:

(1) Public situations structured for meeting strangers, such as

dance halls and discos. These situatons can be very stressful, involving a high risk of rejection and loss of face, especially for male patients. As such, they would not normally be recommended for patients with social skills problems.

(2) Other public situations including bus stops, launderettes, pubs, cafes etc. Here, approaches to strangers can be made in a more discreet fashion, and the risk of overt rejection is greatly reduced. Meeting people in these situations can therefore be more appropriately used as homework tasks.

(3) Private social situations such as a club, private party or a situation within the hospital. Here people have a common bond and may be more receptive to approaches from strangers. The risk of rejection and loss of face is therefore at its lowest in these private contexts, and they are useful starting points for patients to develop skills in meeting strangers.

There are a number of different ways in which a conversation can be opened with a stranger including:

- Questions for help or advice: Do you know how to operate this juke box? I see you're having lasagne, would you recommend it? Is this the right platform for the train for Newtown?
- Offering factual information and seeking reciprocation: Hello, my name is Ricky, what's yours? I'm from Belfast. Where are you from? I'm on my own, do you mind if I join you or are you waiting for someone?
- Giving compliments: That's a lovely dress. I've been admiring your handbag, it's very unusual. I like your hair style.
- Comments about the environment: It's really hot today. I really like this music. It's very smoky in here. The service is very poor tonight.
- Comments about current events: That was a terrible plane crash today. I see taxes have gone up again in the budget. I wish this bus strike would end soon.
- Use of humour: This is more difficult to exemplify, since humour is often situation-specific. It is also more difficult to use effectively, since different people will have different senses of humour. It can, however, be very effective as an ice-breaker.
- The planned accident: The classic example of this is the lady who drops her handkerchief for the gentleman to pick up. Other examples include spilling someone's drink, accidentally tripping

over them, or dropping a handful of small change beside them.
- Being provocative: A certain level of confidence is required before attempting this tactic, since it will not always succeed! Examples would include: I hate to see someone looking so lonely. You have a very closed posture, are you feeling nervous? Do you always drink so much?
- Apparent recognition: Don't I know you from somewhere? I'm sure we've met before. You remind me of X.

Obviously some of these opening strategies bear greater risk than others, and they need to be related to the ability of patients. It should also be remembered that they are merely ice-breakers, and the other skills included in this book will need to be employed successfully in order to keep the conversation going once it has been started (asking questions, giving rewards etc.).

Parting

When we close an interaction, we do not merely stop talking and walk away, and indeed any attempt to close in this way will usually be interpreted as anger or pique. To overcome any such interpretation, we employ a range of closing behaviours in order to ensure that, as the saying goes: 'Parting is such sweet sorrow'. These behaviours are contained within the following functions:

(1) To indicate that closure is about to take place. We use a range of verbal and nonverbal advance indicators to convey the message that we intend to end the interaction in the immediate future. These include: looking at a clock or watch and saying 'Is that the time? I'll have to head off soon'; refusing a drink and saying 'No thanks, I'll have to leave when I've finished this one'. In such situations we often give a reason to suggest that we do not really want to leave, but we have to ('I'll miss my bus', 'The wife will murder me').

(2) To convey commitment to an ongoing relationship. As with greetings, the warmth of partings serves as a barometer for the intensity of the relationship. Two people in love will have an intense parting, as opposed to two people who have just mutually broken off their relationship, where the parting will be brief and cool. Partings between friends will usually involve the whole ritual of smiles, eyebrow flash, head toss, hand signals and appropriate verbalisations (All the best. Safe

home. See you soon). These signals communicate that the interaction has been enjoyable and rewarding, and that the friendship is valued.

(3) To communicate the desire to develop a relationship. This is similar to the previous function, except that here the parting involves someone who has been encountered for the first time. A more overt form of supportiveness is required in order to indicate the wish to pursue interaction in the future. This usually involves providing verbal and nonverbal rewards for the other person, as well as making definite arrangements about meeting again. Closing statements would include: 'I really enjoyed talking to you. Would you like to do this again sometime?' 'I never noticed the time passing. Can I see you again' 'You are really easy to get on with. Will you be here tomorrow?'.

(4) To underline any commitments which have been agreed upon. This ensures that both people are aware of what decisions have been made, and are in accord about who does what. Examples include: 'O.K. I'll get you that book for next week'; 'So you'll get two tickets for the concert'.

(5) To emphasise the particular nature of the relationship between people. Thus, the passionate embrace and goodnight kiss between two lovers will seal the relationship as being close and intimate. The counsellor's summary and arrangement of next appointment highlights the caring nature of his or her relationship with the counsellor, while the firm, brief handshake between two businessmen signals mutual respect within a formal relationship.

(6) To indicate that interaction is definitely at an end. An important function of parting behaviours is to communicate the final episode of the interaction. The terminal exchanges ('Bye' 'So long') coupled with increased inter-personal distance serve to finish smoothly a social encounter. As discussed earlier, the expected duration of separation will influence the choice of behaviours employed during parting. If someone is moving away to another town or another country, there will often be an elaborate and intense parting ritual, because of the reduced likelihood of meeting that person again. Following such a parting, it is often embarrassing for both parties if they do meet again in the near future. For example, someone who is emigrating receives a grand send-off from his office col-

leagues on his last day at work. He then discovers that he has left something behind at the office and returns the next morning to collect it. Under such circumstances, acute embarrassment will be experienced by his colleagues who have already given him their final, intensive parting, and are unsure about how to greet him again. In this context, the closure norms have been broken by the individual returning much too soon after receiving a parting ritual appropriate for a long separation.

Parting is therefore a crucial element of inter-personal interaction. As Phillips (1985) points out:

Think of the behaviours that go into ending or disengaging oneself from an interaction: all the way from hastening away from a person met casually on the street corner to ending a long-term relationship. We have not studied these 'disengaging' kinds of interaction nearly as much as the engaging variety but they are probably equally important.

It is vital for patients to be able to follow the norms associated with greetings and partings. Patients who violate these norms will encounter problems in social interaction. It is therefore important for patients to learn appropriate methods for opening and closing interaction, in a range of situations which they are likely to encounter.

Overview

The three dimensions of social interaction discussed in this chapter are all important areas of study for nurses to implement during SST. Nonverbal communication is a wide area of study, to which appropriate attention should be devoted during training. The way that we behave is often much more important than what we say during social encounters. This is evidenced by the fact that most of us speak for a relatively short period of time each day. It is therefore vital that patients learn about the various aspects of nonverbal communication, and their significance in different contexts. Since nonverbal communication permeates most of the other social skills that have been identified, it is useful to focus upon this aspect initially during SST.

Elements of nonverbal communication play a significant role during self-disclosure, greetings and partings. We provide others with information about ourselves both verbally and nonverbally. Patients must learn how to use self-disclosure effectively, by learning about the norms associated with amount and type of disclosure across social situations. Equally, patients may need to acquire techniques for use in meeting and parting from strangers, to enable them successfully to build up relationships. Knowing what to say to a complete stranger is a problem for many patients, as is knowing how and when to terminate an interaction.

8 COPING SKILLS

This chapter extends the analysis of social skills as presented in Chapter 7. In particular, it is concerned with an overview of those skills essential for coping with everyday social situations. We have included four skill areas in this category, namely asking questions, giving explanations, being assertive and interacting in groups.

Making requests and generally using questions is an important skill in inter-personal interaction. It is a useful technique for opening conversations and for demonstrating interest in others. Patients should therefore be aware of the nature and functions of different types of questions. Explaining is also a very important aspect of social interaction, since it is used to express attitudes, feelings and emotions, as well as to provide others with factual information. The third skill, assertiveness, has been widely employed in programmes of SST, since the ability to stand up for one's rights is something that many patients lack. The final area of study in this chapter is concerned with an examination of some of the factors associated with interacting in groups, another aspect of social interaction that can cause problems for patients. Thus, these four skill areas are important for patients to study during SST.

Asking Questions

The skill of questioning is one of the most important techniques for opening and maintaining conversations with others. The ability to use questions skilfully can enable the patient to cope successfully in a number of social situations, by putting the focus of attention on the other person. The importance of this skill is evidenced by the fact that young children typically ask a barrage of questions in order to gather information about, and make sense of, their environment. Children quickly learn that the best way to learn is to ask! At a more subtle level, however, children also probably discover that questions can be used to manipulate people and situations. For example, the child who asks questions will not only ascertain specific information, but will also receive the attention of others.

In this sense, the questioner is often the controller of a situation. In a selection interview, the interviewer will expect to ask the questions, and will only allow the interviewee to ask questions at set periods (usually at the end of the interview). In classrooms, the teacher asks the vast proportion of questions and will encourage pupils to ask a few, but not too many. Chat-show hosts, detectives, survey interviewers and reporters are other examples of individuals who use questions in order to control interaction. In all of these instances there is a formality attached to the proceedings, which underlines the control exerted by the questioner. In less formal settings, however, questions can be employed to similar advantage. We can find out about others, and keep them talking, by asking questions.

A question can be defined simply as a request for information. Such a request can be verbal or nonverbal. By raising our eyebrows or using a quizzical facial expression we can nonverbally indicate to others that we wish them to provide us with further information. Similarly, by uttering a high-pitched vocalisation ('hmmm?') we can nonverbally 'ask' a question. For the most part, however, we will ask questions verbally, and it is this aspect that should be focused upon during SST. An important function of nonverbal behaviour during verbal questions, however, is to underline the fact that a question is being asked. These nonverbal questioning 'markers' include raising or lowering the vocal inflection on the final syllable of the question, rapidly raising or lowering the eyebrows, head movements, direct eye contact and a pause at the end of the question. All of these behaviours serve to indicate that a request has been made, and a response expected.

Functions of Questions

As Hargie et al (1981) have illustrated, questions serve a large number of functions. In everyday interactions the main functions are as follows:

(1) To obtain information. As the definition indicates, this is the central function of questions. When meeting strangers, questions are an important method for starting a conversation. At this stage in a relationship we often use questions to acquire factual data about other people, so that we can put them in a particular perspective. Questions such as 'What's your name?', and 'Where are you from?', are used to build up

a picture of the other person, as well as to open up possible areas of commonality for discussion.

(2) To express an interest in others. Questions can be employed to communicate to others an interest in them as people. This often happens at the 'chatting up' stage of dating, when both parties ask questions to convey an interest in developing a relationship further.

(3) To ascertain the attitudes and opinions of others. While at the early stage of relationship development questions are used to gather superficial information, as the relationship progresses questions will be utilised to ascertain the beliefs, values and opinions of the other person.

(4) To encourage the other person to participate fully in an inter-action. As mentioned earlier, questioning is a good technique for directing the focus of attention away from oneself and onto others. When used subtly, therefore, questions are potent tools for manipulating a conversation.

(5) To focus attention upon a specific topic. The questioner can, in effect, choose the topic for discussion by raising pertinent questions relating to it. This can be achieved either by ensuring that one's own questions are asked first, or by answering questions asked by the other briefly, and quickly proceeding to follow this up with a different question. In such instances questions can be prefaced by phrases such as: 'There's some-thing I've been meaning to ask you ...' or 'I'd be interested in your views on ...'

These five functions are obviously very important during social encounters. For this reason, patients should be encouraged to develop their repertoire of questions. Not knowing what to say is a problem often cited by patients, and this can be partially overcome by the use of questions coupled with listening and rewarding behaviours (see Chapter 9). Patients should, therefore, be aware of how different types of questions can influence the flow of conver-sation.

Types of Question

A number of different types of classifications of questions have been identified by psychologists and linguists. We will focus upon those classifications that have direct relevance to the types of situ-ation which patients are likely to experience.

Closed/open.   One of the most common distinctions is between
closed questions and open questions. This distinction is based
upon the degree of scope that the question allows the respondent
in choosing how to answer. As the name suggests, closed questions
place restrictions upon the respondent by closing down the number
of expected options available. The respondent may, of course,
refuse to accept these restrictions and pursue other options. Thus,
to the question 'What's your name?' the respondent could reply
'It's none of your business!' In most interactions, however, it is eti-
quette to accept the restrictions, especially if the respondent wishes
to maintain a relationship with the questioner. Closed questions
are categorised as such by the nature of the question, rather than
by the response evoked. For example the question, 'Have you been
waiting here long?' can be satisfactorily answered 'Yes' or 'No',
and is therefore closed. At the same time, it is possible that the
respondent may answer by giving a detailed account of how fed up
he or she is waiting, how poor the service is, and so on. Regardless
of which response is given, we would classify the question as
closed. A question is said to be closed if it falls within one of the
following three categories:

(1) The selection question. Here the respondent is expected to
    choose one from two or more alternatives. This type of
    question is also referred to as forced-choice. Examples would
    include: 'Do you prefer tea or coffee?' 'Would you like to go
    to the cinema or to the theatre?'
(2) The yes/no question. This question simply requires a 'yes' or
    'no' as the answer. For example: 'Do you smoke?' 'Are you
    Irish?' 'Would you like another drink?'
(3) The identification question. In this case, the respondent is
    expected to identify a piece of factual information and provide
    this as the answer to the question. This may involve the recall
    of information ('Where were you born?' 'What is your maiden
    name?'), the identification of current information ('What time
    is it?' 'What age are you?') or future events ('How are you
    getting home?' 'Where are you going on holiday?').

Closed questions are easy to answer, and for this reason they
are quite often used during initial encounters, when factual information is being exchanged. They do not, however, encourage any
length or depth of response, and open questions are therefore

more appropriate for this purpose. Open questions allow the respondent a greater degree of freedom in deciding how to respond. In other words, the response is left open to the respondent. Open questions are broad in nature and require more than a one or two-word answer. However, some open questions will place more restrictions on respondents than others, and in this sense open questions can be regarded as forming a continuum from the very open to the slightly open. Consider the following sequence:

(A) 'What do you do in your spare time?'
(B) 'What do you do in the evenings?'
(C) 'What do you do on Saturday evenings?'
(D) 'What did you do last Saturday evening?'

In this sequence, the focus of the questions has gradually narrowed from the initial very open question (A) to the more restricted open question (D).

Open questions are useful for encouraging maximum participation. Indeed, the available research evidence would tend to suggest that responses to open questions are about three times as long in duration as responses to closed questions. To date, little research has been conducted into patterns of questioning among social inadequates, and it would be interesting to ascertain both whether they use questions as frequently as more socially skilled individuals, and whether they tend to concentrate on closed questions. Certainly, the potential benefits of open questions should be highlighted for patients during SST.

Probing.   A probe is a follow-up question used to build upon an initial response. It is used to encourage respondents to expand upon an answer by providing further related information. This can be achieved by using a variety of types of probing questions as follows:

(1) Clarification probes. These are employed to elicit a clearer response in a situation where there is some ambiguity about what the respondent has just said. In other words, clarification is being sought by questions such as: 'What do you mean?' 'Could you explain that?' or 'In what ways?'
(2) Justification probes. These are used to seek a justification from

the respondent with regard to what he or she has just said, by giving reasons for the response. Examples would include: 'Why do you say that?' 'How do you know?' or 'How did you come to that conclusion?'

(3) Extension probes. Here the purpose is to get the respondent simply to provide further information by extending their initial response. This can be achieved by asking: 'And then what happened?' 'Can you remember anything else about it?', or by saying 'Tell me more'.

(4) Exemplification probes. This type of probe is used to request the respondent to provide specific examples of that which they have been describing. This can often help to put the respondent's thoughts into perspective, by seeking a concrete example of what may have been a somewhat vague statement. Included here would be questions such as 'Can you give me an example?' 'Can you think of an exact instance of where this occurred?' or 'What type of ...?'

(5) Accuracy probes. These questions enable the questioner to check the accuracy of a response, and allow respondents to adjust or revise their initial answers accordingly. Examples would be: 'Are you sure about that?' 'You are certain it was him?' or 'Is this definite?'

(6) Echo probes. Sometimes referred to as 'parroting', this simply involves repeating, in an inquisitive fashion, the last few words uttered by the respondent. We often use these in social interaction, but if they are over-used they can be counterproductive, since they will be viewed by the respondent as artificial. Examples of echo probes are included in the following sequence:

A. I don't enjoy going to the theatre but I like going to the cinema.
Q. You like going to the cinema?
A. Yes, it seems more realistic. Yet I haven't been to the movies for over five years.
Q. Five years?!

(7) Nonverbal probes. As discussed earlier, nonverbal behaviours can be used to request information, and these are mainly employed as probes. Included here would be appropriate paralanguage to accompany expressions such as 'Really?!'

'Never?!' or 'Ohh?' Other forms of nonverbal probes would include raising or lowering the eyebrows fully, together with head movements and eye contact.

These are the main forms of probe which can be employed during social interaction. Probes are of value in that they indicate both attention to and interest in the respondent. Patients should learn when and how to employ probing questions to best effect. In particular, they should be made aware of the danger of over-using probes in an interrogative, demanding fashion on the one hand, and of not using any probes at all on the other.

Affective Questions. These questions focus specifically on the affective domain, namely the emotions, attitudes and feelings of the respondent. This is a crucial facet of interpersonal communication, and one that patients should be encouraged to explore with others. The exchange of feelings usually increases and deepens as a relationship develops. At an early stage, such exchanges tend to be superficial, with affective questions such as: 'Do you like this music?' or 'Did you enjoy the film?' It is only later that questions such as 'Do you love me?' will be asked. Patients should learn to develop the skill of asking appropriate affective questions in various situations.

Leading Questions. These are questions that lead the respondent towards an expected response. Two main types are relevant for patients:

(1) Conversational leads. These are frequently used during conversations to stimulate the flow of conversation. They should anticipate correctly the response the other person would be likely to make, and are therefore a positive method for showing common understanding. Such leads include 'Isn't that a terrible day?', 'It's really cold in here, isn't it?'.

(2) Simple leads. These are questions that are intended to lead the respondent in the direction the questioner wants him or her to go, regardless of the answer which the respondent is likely to give. They therefore place pressure on the respondent to agree, and can be off-putting for this reason. Examples are: 'Wouldn't you agree that abortion is murder?' 'Surely you don't support those awful socialists?' 'Aren't the social

security benefits in this country already far too high?' Interestingly, however, it has been found that asking a simple lead which is blatantly wrong can provoke a lengthy response, since this places the respondent in the position of expert *vis-à-vis* the misinformed questioner. Thus saying: 'You're from Wales. Isn't that one of the few regions to escape the increase in unemployment?', would probably encourage a detailed response from a Welshman!

Both of these types of leading question can therefore be gainfully employed in social interaction. With practice, patients can learn when they are appropriate. At the same time, there are risks associated with both leads. Conversational leads that are inaccurate will convey a lack of shared understanding (e.g. saying 'Isn't this lovely weather?' when the rain is pouring down!). Similarly, the unskilled use of simple leads will give an impression of lack of concern or interest in the respondent.

Related Aspects of Questioning

Some behaviours related to the skill of questioning can influence the outcome of an interaction.

Structuring: This involves informing a respondent in advance what questions are going to be asked. This is a useful strategy when making enquiries, since it allows the respondent to 'tune in' to the questioner's frame of reference. The respondent will thereby realise what the goals of the questioner are, in advance of the forthcoming questions. Examples of structuring are: 'Excuse me, I wonder could you give me some information about my entitlement to housing benefits? I've just become unemployed and want to know if I am eligible ...' 'I'm a stranger here and I'm in need of some help to find my way to one or two places. Could you help ...'

Pausing: It is possible to use pauses to good effect before a question is asked, after the question has been asked, and after a response has been obtained. A brief pause prior to posing a question allows time for thoughtful phrasing. Pausing after asking a question and after receiving an answer has been found to encourage respondents to develop their answers fully (Hargie et al, 1981). Such pauses put subtle pressure on the respondent to participate.

Prompting: This is the technique that is used to encourage a respondent to give an adequate answer, following a failure to do so, to a previous question. Different forms of prompt can be employed depending upon the hypothesised cause of the inadequate response. These include restating the same question, rephrasing the question, asking a simpler question or providing a clue to help the respondent to focus upon the desired aspect.

In addition to these positive aspects of questioning, there are some practices to be avoided. These include either flooding the other person with questions or not asking any questions at all. Another common failing is asking multiple questions. A multiple question comprises two or more separate questions strung together (e.g. 'Are you on your own? Don't I know you? Would you like a drink?'). This is a specific form of flooding which only serves to confuse the respondent, and patients should be encouraged to ask one question at a time. Finally, answering one's own questions is another indicator of lack of skill, and is something that patients should learn to refrain from doing. Most of these negative aspects tend to be caused by nervousness, and with increased practice and experience they can be overcome.

Topics for Questioning

Knowing what to ask questions about is as important as knowing how to ask questions skilfully, and so attention should also be devoted to this area during SST. Trower et al (1978) suggest four main topic areas for questions:

(1) Anything the other person has recently been involved in
(2) Aspects of the other person's life including: work, home, travel, hobbies and social activities
(3) Things that both people have in common, including the immediate environment, TV, cinema, pubs, cars, hi-fi, friends and acquaintances
(4) Current local and national events, including news, gossip, sport, personalities, politics and forthcoming attractions.

During SST it is useful to allow patients to practise their questioning skills using a range of situations they are likely to encounter. This may include asking for help, advice or information, opening a conversation with a stranger, maintaining a conversation, or dating. The objective here is not to provide patients with a set list of pre-arranged questions for every situation, but rather to boost their confidence in their own questioning ability.

Explaining

Giving explanations forms an important part of inter-personal communication. In order to convey to others our attitudes, beliefs, opinions, thoughts, ideas and experiences we have to use this skill. The ability to explain in a succinct, lucid and coherent fashion is therefore a central facet of social skill. It is also an area in which many patients will experience problems. Common failings here include either being too verbose and giving long, meandering explanations which provide details about even the smallest, inconsequential aspects on the one hand, or being monosyllabic and not explaining even the most crucial aspects on the other. The inability to follow a logical structure is another reason for lack of success in explaining, as is a lack of clarity of speech.

In everyday parlance, the verb 'to explain' has two meanings, 'a meaning which emphasises the *intention* of the explainer, and a meaning which emphasises the *success* of the explanation' (Turney et al, 1976). It therefore makes sense to say 'I explained it to him but he was too stupid to understand'. However, for our purposes we will not use this meaning, but will rather use a definition that underlines success rather than intention, namely that to explain is to give understanding to another. This is a more acceptable approach from the perspective of social interaction, in that it gives prime consideration to the effects of the explanation upon the listener.

Functions of Explanations

The skill of explaining serves a number of functions in social interaction. These are as follows:

(1) To provide others with factual information. This type of explanation would be given in response to questions such as 'Can you tell me how to get to the railway station?' or 'How do I go about getting my car tax?' No great depth of explanation is required here, but rather a simple exposition of the main elements involved.
(2) To convey one's attitudes, feelings or emotions. This is an

important function of explanations for many patients, who should learn not only to identify their affective state, but also to communicate this to others. The inability to recognise and express one's feelings can lead to frustration and inappropriate social behaviour.

(3) To relate personal experiences. A great deal of social interaction is taken up with explaining to others where we have been and what we have seen or done. The giving and receiving of such information forms an important part of inter-personal encounters, and it is important that patients develop the ability to give coherent, meaningful accounts of their experiences.

(4) To express opinions. Another facet of social interaction is the expression of one's own views and the debating of these views with others. Patients should therefore be encouraged to develop the ability to state their opinions succinctly yet forcibly.

(5) To demonstrate a technique. On some occasions it is necessary to explain by actually giving a demonstration. If asked how to operate a juke-box or a video-recorder, it is much easier to explain the operation by offering a demonstration and showing the person what to do.

(6) To give a justification for an action. This type of explanation would be necessary when returning faulty goods to a shop, and indeed in all situations where we are asked to justify why we are doing something. In such instances it is vital to be able to give valid, rational reasons for our actions.

These six functions of explaining underline the importance of this skill for patients, who should be given an opportunity to develop and refine their explaining skills during SST.

Presentation

The presentation of an explanation will be influenced by the extent to which the person is able to plan in advance. Most explanations in everyday interaction are of a spontaneous nature, and cannot really be planned in advance. However, in some cases it is possible to prepare an explanation and where this is so, the person should:

(1) Carefully decide what the main aspects of the explanation are
(2) Determine how these aspects should be linked
(3) Where appropriate, consider how any views being expressed in

the explanation can be supported
(4) Estimate what views may be put forward by others, and how these may be dealt with
(5) Relate the explanation to the background knowledge and ability of the recipient.

Whether or not it is possible to plan an explanation, a number of factors will influence the extent to which it is successful. Some of these can be summarised by comparing a good explanation to a good bikini, in that both should be brief and appealing, should cover the essentials, and certain parts should stick out!

Brevity.   Explanations that are too long will not usually be successful since listeners will tend to 'switch off'. On the other hand, it is necessary to provide enough detail to make the explanation meaningful. Patients should therefore attempt to achieve a balanced length when giving explanations.

Appeal.   Good explanations will be appealing to the listener who should be interested in what is being covered. Thus, the explanation should be tailored to suit the interests, age, sex, and so on of the listener. For example, most young females are not really interested in the intricacies of motor cycles, and so explanations on this topic would not really have appeal for them!

Essential Features.   In order to cover the central features, it is necessary to provide emphasis in an explanation. Emphasis is the process whereby the core details are underlined while more peripheral information is kept in the background (in other words, certain parts stick out!). Once these core details have been identified, they can be emphasised both verbally and nonverbally. Nonverbal emphasis can be achieved by use of hands, face, arms and voice delivery. Movement of parts of the body to give emphasis and stimulate attention is referred to as speaker animation. All good public speakers are aware of the value of appearing animated and enthusiastic when delivering speeches. This can be witnessed by observing politicians, actors or even comedians appearing in public. If the speaker appears dull and disinterested he is not likely to fire any enthusiasm in the audience. By moving hands, arms, body and changing facial expressions, the speaker can both stimulate attention and provide emphasis. For example, by holding up three fingers and saying 'there are three main points', by using gestures to illustrate shape or movement, and by laughing to underline a humorous episode, the speaker can convey the important elements.

Changes in vocal pattern are also of immense value. By raising or lowering the volume of the voice, by altering the speed of delivery, by changing pitch or tone, and by employing mimicry, the speaker can both hold attention and give emphasis to particular points. However, this can be one of the most difficult areas for patients to change. We tend to be very self-conscious about deliberately altering our speech styles, and can find trying to do so very disconcerting too. Nevertheless, it is possible to effect changes, and the outcome can be well worth the effort. One famous politician when asked whether his powerful skills of oratory came naturally or were developed by him, replied: 'Naturally. I have worked so hard at it that naturally I improved!' Patients who speak in a dull, flat, monotone should certainly be encouraged to develop a less boring pattern of delivery.

Emphasis can also be achieved by verbal techniques. An example of this is the use of verbal cueing to highlight specific aspects of an explanation. Verbal cues are words or phrases which serve to underline important parts, and would include phrases such as: 'What you must remember is ...'; 'Now this is important ...'; 'What all this adds up to ...'; or words such as 'main', 'central', 'crucial'. The use of such cueing techniques has been found to increase significantly the ability of listeners to remember the information immediately following the cues. Another form of verbal emphasis is the use of planned repetition. Again, this is a method used by all good public speakers, who want to ensure that they get their core message across. By repeating the main points at intervals throughout an explanation, it is more likely to be remembered. However, there will always be an optimum amount of repetition, beyond which any benefits gained will be quickly lost. While there is truth in the maxim 'Something worth saying is worth repeating', something repeated *ad nauseum* will evidently be counterproductive.

Verbal and nonverbal techniques for achieving emphasis should be practised by patients during SST, since they are central to successful explanation. As Turney et al (1973) point out: 'At one level they simply attract attention; at another they help convey meaning; and at another they stimulate interest.'

Fluency. People rated as being skilled at giving explanations are fluent speakers who can avoid using too many 'ums' and 'ers' during their presentations. When we are anxious we tend to make more speech errors both of the latter type, and of what are referred to as 'non-ah' errors, namely stuttering, stammering, slips of the tongue, unfinished sentences and sentence changes (starting a sentence and then changing it in midstream). These speech dysfluencies will detract greatly from the success of an explanation. As mentioned in Chapter 7, if these dysfluencies are of a severe nature they may require the intervention of a speech therapist. If, however, they are a result of social anxiety they can usually be reduced following appropriate practice and feedback during SST.

Structuring. As discussed earlier in this chapter, structuring involves informing someone in advance of what is about to be said. Thus, before giving an explanation, it is useful to prepare the listener for that which is to follow. This allows people to set themselves and 'tune in' to the ensuing information. Examples of structuring would include: 'I must tell you what I did last night ...'; 'I think I should explain why I am here ...' 'Wait until you hear about ...'

Pausing. The use of pauses can facilitate explanations, especially for those patients who may be inclined to rush through material at a great speed. Pauses serve to punctuate the delivery, they allow time for the listener to assimilate information, and they permit the speaker to gather their thoughts before presenting them. In this way, the use of pauses can help to reduce the number of speech dysfluencies. At the same time, pauses need to be of an appropriate length (usually not longer than 3 or 4 seconds) during social interaction, since longer 'pregnant' pauses can cause embarrassment for both speaker and listener.

Avoiding Vagueness. An explanation should be clear and coherent so that the listener is not left in any doubt about exactly what is meant. The explainer should be as succinct as possible to avoid confusing the listener with unnecessary information. He should also try to link each part of the explanation, so that there is a logical progression of details, and the listener knows who or what is being referred to at any particular time. The use of what Turney et al (1976) refer to as 'indeterminate expressions' have been found to be associated with lack of success in explanation, and should therefore be avoided. Such expressions would include 'kind of thing', 'are not necessarily', 'a bunch of', 'about as much as', 'was not quite', 'they say that'. Obviously, we all use one or more of these expressions on occasion, and it is their continued, sustained use that is to be avoided.

Language. As discussed in Chapter 4, our use of language varies from one situation to another, and indeed the ability to alter the language used across situations is an indicator of social skill. Patients may need to learn to tailor the language used in their explanations to suit the variety of situations they are likely to encounter. The choice of vocabulary will depend upon the age and ability of the listener as well as the context within which the explanation occurs. Thus, terms used when explaining to adults will not usually be understood by young infants, while the type of language acceptable in a working man's club may not be appropriate at a selection interview!

Examples. When explaining new or unfamiliar material, it is often useful to employ examples to illustrate points being made. This helps to anchor the new material within a framework that is more familiar to the listener. This is a technique widely used by the media; for example, when explaining the details of a new Budget, radio, TV and newspapers will give examples of how exactly it will affect people of different incomes and different circumstances. This helps to make the explanation 'come alive' for the recipient. Where examples are used they should be relevant to the listener's experience, meaningful in relation to the explanation, specific and concrete, and as brief as possible. In everyday interaction most examples will be verbal, although it may be possible to give written examples (e.g. a diagram of a building) or to use some form of pictorial example (e.g. a photograph). Examples are commonly used to support arguments and underline points being made. For example during debates about the pros and cons of legalised abortion, supporters of abortion frequently cite the case of the woman who has been brutally raped, whereas opponents give the example of the female who views abortion as just another form of birth control. Thus, it is important for patients to develop the ability to provide relevant and appropriate examples during explanations. A final type of example is an actual demonstration.

When asked for information about how to operate a piece of equipment (e.g. a juke box) it can be simpler actually to show the other person what to do rather than try to explain the process verbally.

Feedback. The definition of explaining given earlier implicitly emphasised the crucial role of feedback, since if we wish to give understanding to another we need to ascertain to what extent we have been successful in so doing. By obtaining feedback from listeners we are able to gauge how far we need to alter our explanations to make them more comprehensible. Without such feedback, our explanations would be more haphazard, hit-or-miss affairs. As discussed in Chapter 4, patients need to be sensitive to the inter-personal cues being emitted by others, and use these to guide their own behaviour. During explanations, feedback can be obtained both verbally and nonverbally. By scanning the nonverbal behaviour of the listener it is possible to estimate whether he is confused (frowns, raised eyebrows, 'blank looks'), bored (less eye contact, dull facial expression, yawns) or attentive (good eye contact, head nods, smiles). On the basis of this feedback the explanations may be simplified, shortened or expanded respectively. Feedback can also be obtained verbally by asking the listener questions. Any possible embarrassment here can be overcome by prefacing such feedback questions with phrases such as 'I'm not sure whether I've explained that very well ...' or 'That's probably about as clear as mud ...'.

Assertiveness

Assertiveness as an area of study has a long history within SST. Indeed, as Kelly (1982) points out: 'until somewhat recently, the terms "assertion training" and "social-skills training" were often used in interchangeable fashion; it was not recognised that assertiveness represents one specific kind of interpersonal competency'. This ambiguity is not really surprising when some definitions of assertiveness are examined. For example, Lazarus (1971) regarded assertiveness as comprising four main components, namely the ability to:

(1) Refuse request

(2) Ask for favours and make requests
(3) Express positive and negative feelings
(4) Initiate, continue and terminate general conversations

It is obvious that this definition of assertiveness is very wide, encompassing almost all forms of human interaction! Dissatisfaction with this approach has led to a more focused approach to the study of assertion, based upon the specific aspect of standing up for one's rights. This latter interpretation is the one given by most dictionaries, and the perspective held by most laymen, and it is the view that we will discuss here. Thus, an appropriate definition of assertive behaviour is that it is behaviour which 'enables a person to act in his or her own best interests, to stand up for herself or himself without undue anxiety, to express honest feelings comfortably, or to exercise personal rights without denying the rights of others' (Alberti and Emmons, 1982). In like vein, Liberman et al (1975) define assertiveness in terms of the defence of personal rights, self confidence, the ability to express feelings, goal achievement, and the exercise of choice. These two definitions embrace the main elements of assertiveness.

Assertiveness, Aggression and Nonassertiveness

In order to understand fully the concept of assertiveness, it is necessary to distinguish this style of responding from two other styles, namely aggression and nonassertiveness. Consider the following three responses to a situation in which someone is asked for a loan of a book that they did not wish to lend:

(1) 'No. Why don't you buy your own damn books!'
(2) 'Um ... How long would you need it for? It's just that, ah, I might need it for an assignment. But if it wasn't for long'
(3) I'm sorry. I'd like to help you out, but I bought this book so that I would always have it to refer to, so I never lend it to anyone.'

Here the first response is aggressive, the second nonassertive and the third assertive. Alberti and Emmons (1975) distinguish between these three styles of responding as follows:

Aggressive Responses. These involve threatening or violating the rights of the other person. Here the person answers before the other is finished speaking, talks loudly and abusively, glares at the other person, speaks 'past' the issue (accusing, blaming, demeaning), vehemently states feelings and opinions, values himself above others, and hurts others to avoid hurting himself. The objective here is to win, regardless of the other person.

Nonassertive Responses.   These involve expressing oneself in such a self-effacing, apologetic manner that one's thoughts, feelings and rights can easily be ignored. In this 'cap in hand' style, the person hesitates, speaks softly, looks away, avoids issues, agrees regardless of his own feelings, does not express opinions, values himself 'below' others, and hurts himself to avoid any chance of hurting others. The objective here is to appease others and avoid conflict at any cost.

Assertive Responses.   These involve standing up for oneself, yet taking the other person into consideration. The assertive style involves answering spontaneously, speaking with a conversational yet firm tone and volume, looking at the other person, addressing the main issue, openly expressing personal feelings and opinions, valuing oneself equal to others, and hurting neither oneself nor others. The objective here is to try to ensure fair play for everyone.

Of these three styles, assertiveness is usually the most appropriate. Aggressive individuals may initially get their own way by browbeating others, but will then be disliked and avoided. Alternatively, this style may provoke a similar response from others, with the danger that escalating verbal aggression will lead to overt physical aggression. Nonassertive individuals, on the other hand, will often be viewed by others as weak, 'mealy mouthed' creatures who can be easily manipulated, and as a result non-assertive people will frequently express dissatisfaction with their lives, owing to a failure to attain personal goals. Assertive individuals, however, tend to derive more satisfaction from their dealings with others, since they feel more in control of their own lives, and achieve their goals more often. They also will obtain more respect from those with whom they interact.

Most people will have a general style of interacting, whether it be assertive, nonassertive or aggressive. At the same time, individuals may be assertive in some situations, yet nonassertive or aggressive in others. Thus, it is necessary for the nurse to ascertain in exactly which situations a patient finds difficulty in being assertive, and then it is possible to tackle these specific problems during SST. There may be some patients who have a consistent pattern of nonassertiveness (generalised nonassertiveness) and here the problems of remediation are much greater. It should also be remembered that there may be a variety of reasons for a patient being nonassertive, some of which are more valid than others. The main reasons for not being assertive include:

(1) Mistaking assertiveness for aggression. Some patients confuse these two styles of responding in such a way that they believe that standing up for their rights will be seen as aggressive behaviour by others. This problem is especially pronounced amongst some female patients who may perceive assertiveness as being aggressive and masculine, and view their role as being always nonassertive.

(2) Not wanting to lose friends, by being seen as pushy. Once a nonassertive style has been developed, it becomes resistant to change, since people are worried that if they change to an assertive style they will lose their friends or spouse. Patients need to learn that, when used appropriately, assertive behaviour will usually be accepted by those with whom they interact.

(3) Wanting to avoid any possible confrontation. Here the person wishes to settle for an easy, trouble-free life and so is prepared to forego almost any personal rights in order to avoid strife. The problem is that people who adopt such a totally sub-missive style will tend to be used and abused by others and are often unhappy. Patients with this outlook need to learn that their nonassertive style will cause them many more problems than would assertiveness.

(4) Mistaking assertiveness for bad manners. Some patients may feel that it is not polite to assert themselves. They may have been brought up under a very strict regime by parents in which as children they were 'seen and not heard', and learned in school that the quiet child who did as it was told was most approved of by the teacher. It can then be difficult in later life to overcome this residue of parental and educational upbringing. Patients who suffer from this misapprehension need to learn that being assertive does not negate politeness.

(5) Not being confident in carrying things off. Many patients will

feel a strong desire to stand up for their rights, but have not learned how to do so and are therefore lacking in confidence. For these patients, training in assertiveness should form an important component of SST, and they should be given ample opportunity to role-play situations in which they wish to be more assertive.

(6) Mistaking nonassertion for being helpful. Some people will be viewed by others as 'easy touches', in terms of borrowing money, etc., since they are always ready to be helpful. Obviously, there comes a time when being helpful develops into being used, and patients need to learn not only to be able to draw the line between these two, but also actually to resist unreasonable requests by responding assertively.

(7) Seeing that someone is in a difficult situation. If you are in a busy restaurant and you know that a new waitress has just been employed, you are more likely to overlook certain issues, such as someone who came in later being served before you. Here, it is appropriate to be nonassertive, since personal rights are not deliberately being denied, and to be assertive may cause undue stress to the other person.

(8) Interacting with a highly sensitive individual. If by being assertive someone is liable to burst into floods of tears, or physically attack you, it may be wise to be nonassertive, especially if the encounter is 'one-off'.

(9) Manipulating others. Some females will deliberately employ a helpless style in order to achieve their goals, for example to encourage a male to change a flat tyre on their car. Males may do likewise. For example, if stopped by police following a minor traffic misdemeanour it may be wise to be nonassertive ('I'm terribly sorry, officer, but I've just bought this car'). Such behaviour is more likely to achieve positive benefits.

Types of Assertiveness

A number of different types of assertive behaviour can be employed. Lange and Jakubowski (1976) identify five types of assertiveness:

Basic Assertion. This involves a simple direct expression of standing up for personal rights, beliefs, feelings or opinions. For example, when interrupted a basic assertion expression would be: 'Excuse me, I would like to finish what I was saying'.

Empathic Assertion.   This type of assertion conveys some sensitivity to the other person, by making a statement that conveys some recognition of the other person's situation or feelings before making the assertive statement. Thus, an empathic assertion to an interruption might be: 'I know you are keen to get your views across, but I would like to finish what I was saying'.

Escalating Assertion.   Here the individual begins by making a minimal assertion response, and, if the other person fails to respond to this, gradually increases or escalates the degree of assertiveness employed. Two females having a quiet drink in a bar may use the following escalating assertive responses to a man who keeps interrupting them and offers to buy them drinks:

(A) Thanks for the offer, but we are just here for a quiet drink and a personal chat
(B) No thanks, as I've already said we don't want any drink. We just want to be left alone
(C) Look, would you please go away and stop annoying us. If you don't I will have to complain to the management.

Confrontive Assertion.   This is used when someone's words contradict their actions, and involves clearly telling the person what he said he would do, and what he actually did. The speaker then expresses what he now wants. An example would be: 'You said you would return my books by Tuesday. It is now Thursday and you still haven't returned them. I would like you to get them for me now so that I can do my assignment'.

I-language Assertion.   Here the speaker objectively describes the behaviour of the other person, how this affects the speaker's life or feelings and why the other person should change his behaviour. In the case of being interrupted, an I-language assertive response would be: 'You know, this is the fourth time you've interrupted me in the past few minutes. This makes me feel that you aren't interested in what I am saying, and I feel a bit hurt and annoyed. I would like you to let me finish what I want to say.'

Linehan and Egan (1979) distinguish between a direct and an indirect style of assertiveness. They argue that a direct, unambiguous assertive style may not always be most effective, especially for those individuals for whom it is important to be liked and regarded positively by others. Rather, a more ambiguous, indirect style of response seems more appropriate in some instances (despite the fact that most texts recommend a direct style). An example of these two styles can be seen in relation to the following question:

> *Question:* Could you lend me that new LP you bought yesterday?
> *Direct:* No, I never lend my LPs to anyone.
> *Indirect:* Oh, you mean The Oceans — You know, I'm still trying to get a chance to sit down and listen to it at length myself. I usually take ages listening to a new LP.

However, Lineham and Egan also point out that the direct style can be less abrasive if turned into a complex-direct style. This approach would involve the use of an embellishment associated with a refusal. They identify five main embellishments that can be employed: empathy, helplessness, apology, flattery and outright lying (although this one would need to be used with caution). The idea here is to 'soften' the refusal and so maintain a relationship. Thus, using this style a response to the above question might be:

> *Complex-Direct*: I know you would look after it really well, but I've recently had three LPs that I lent ruined, so I've just had to make the general decision never to lend my LPs to anyone again. That way I hope no-one will feel personally offended.

Rakos (1986) points out that assertiveness is usually required when making a refusal, requesting other people to change their behaviour, or expressing an unpopular or different opinion. In all three cases, the individual will have to be assertive in order to ensure his rights are not violated. Rakos also points out that it is useful to conceive of assertion as the mid-point of a continuum of responses ranging from nonassertion at one end to aggression at the other. He identified four main components of assertiveness:

Content.   The actual content of an assertive response should include both an expression of rights and a statement placing this expression of rights within the context of socially responsible and appropriate behaviour. Rakos identifies five possible accompanying statements. We will illustrate these in relation to a refusal to go with a friend to the cinema:

(A) An explanation for the necessity to assert oneself — 'I can't go tonight. I have an essay to finish for tomorrow morning'
(B) An empathic statement recognising the other person's feelings — 'I can't go tonight, I know you are disappointed'
(C) Praise for the other person — 'I can't go tonight, but it was very kind of you to ask'
(D) An apology for any resulting consequences — 'I can't go tonight. I'm sorry that you have no-one else to go with'
(E) An attempt to identify a mutually acceptable compromise — 'I can't go tonight. How would you feel about waiting until Friday night?'

Nonverbal Responses. From a review of research, Rakos recommends:

- Medium levels of eye contact (too much is associated with aggression, too little with nonassertion)
- Avoidance of inappropriate facial expressions (uncontrolled, twitching mouth; wrinkled forehead; animated, moving eyebrows)
- Smooth steady use of gestures while speaking, yet inconspicuous while listening
- Upright posture
- Direct body orientation to the other person
- Appropriate paralinguistics, including a short response latency, a medium duration of response length, good fluency of speech, medium volume (again too loud is aggressive, too soft nonassertive), medium inflection, and increased firmness.

Process. The *way* in which responses are carried out can be crucial to success. Thus the correct timing of vocalisations and nonverbal responses is vital. Stimulus control skills are also important; these refer to manipulation of the environment or the other person, to make the assertive response more successful (e.g. saying you need time to think over a request, or requesting a move to a suitable location prior to being assertive). Rakos also emphasises the need to begin with the minimal effective assertive response, and only escalate the degree of assertion as required.

Covert elements. This refers to the influence of thoughts, ideas and feelings upon the ability to be assertive. Rakos (1986) highlights the following covert aspects:

(1) Knowledge. In order to be assertive, it is necessary to know what an assertive response actually entails.
(2) Self-instructions. This refers to those covert behaviour-guiding self-statements which we employ when making decisions about which responses to carry out. Nonassertive individuals tend to use self-statements such as 'He will not like me if I refuse', rather than 'I have a right to refuse'.
(3) Expectancies. Nonassertive people will negatively evaluate the potential outcomes of being assertive, and will view their ability to be assertive as being poor.
(4) Beliefs. Nonassertiveness can result from mistaken beliefs. For example, a female may believe that a wife should always do as her husband tells her.
(5) Social perception. Nonassertive people tend to perceive the behaviour of others inaccurately (e.g. perceiving unreasonable requests as being reasonable).

These covert elements of patients will need to be explored by the nurse at some stage of SST, since inappropriate thoughts, beliefs or feelings may well be the cause of nonassertiveness for many patients.

Fry (1983) identifies three types of assertiveness which she refers to as 'protective skills', and which are a form of verbal defence commonly used against manipulation, nagging or rudeness. The first of these skills is the *broken record* where the person simply makes an assertive statement and keeps repeating this statement until it is accepted by the other person. For example, to repeated pleas for a loan the individual may just keep saying 'No, I'm not going to give you any money'. The second protective skill is known as *fogging*, wherein the person appears to accept negative criticism without changing his behaviour. An example of a fogging sequence would be:

A: That jacket is too big for you
B: Yes. It probably is
A: It doesn't match your trousers
B: No. It probably doesn't

A: You really look a mess
B: You're probably right.

The idea here is that eventually the other person will become tired of getting no real response to the criticisms and will eventually give up.

It should be realised that these two skills are basic forms of assertion which should really only be used as a form of protection from prolonged or unwarranted criticism. They are not intended as general methods for expressing one's rights. The third type of skill listed by Fry is that of *metalevel assertion* whereby someone who realizes that a solution is unlikely, suggests that wider perspectives should be considered rather than specific issues. One example of this approach, of moving from the particular to the general, would be where a woman involved in an argument with her husband says 'We obviously are not going to agree about this, and I think this is typical of what is happening to our whole relationship'.

Finally, it is useful to alert patients to some possible negative reactions of other people to their new-found assertiveness. Alberti and Emmons (1975) identify four such reactions:

(1) Back-biting. Making statements behind the patient's back, which they may make sure the patient overhears (e.g. 'Who does he think he is?' 'All of a sudden he's now a big fellow').
(2) Aggression. Other people may try to negate the patient's right to assert himself by using threatening, aggressive behaviour.
(3) Over-apologising. Some people may feel they have caused offence and as a result apologise profusely.
(4) Revenge-seeking. The assertiveness may be accepted, but the person will have hidden resentment and a desire to get their own back.

Patients should be prepared for any such reactions and learn how to handle them as an integral part of SST.

These elements of assertiveness comprise an important aspect of inter-personal competence, which should enable patients to cope more effectively during social encounters. In particular, the skilled use of assertive responses will help patients to:

• Effectively communicate their own position on any issue
• Ensure that their rights are not violated

- Withstand unreasonable requests from others
- Cope with refusals from others
- Make reasonable requests of others
- Change the behaviour of others towards them

Interacting in Groups

For most patients, interacting in groups will pose serious problems, and where a social skills deficit exists, this can be an especially marked area of difficulty. At the same time, it is inevitable that patients will have to participate, to some extent, in the presence of others. Groups are important in our society since they serve five important functions as below.

They Help us to Achieve Certain Goals or Fulfil Specific Needs.   Most of our needs are, in fact, met through the operation of groups. If we examine Maslow's hierarchy of needs (Chapter 4), it can be seen that in our society we satisfy needs at each level by forming relevant groups. Thus, there are groups concerned with the production and distribution of food (physiological needs) or with the protection of citizens (safety needs).

They Help us to Gain a Sense of Identity.   Membership of groups provides us with a sense of who we are, and participating in a particular group can strengthen this feeling of identity. Thus, a devout Catholic may attend Mass on a regular basis to underline this aspect of personal identity. Similarly a husband and wife may wish to have a child in order to achieve a family group identity.

They Enable us to Interact with Others whom we Perceive to be Similar.   By joining a women's rights group, a Christian fellowship group, or a vegetarian society, the individual will know in advance that other members of the group will hold similar views on at least one important issue. The chances of being assimilated into the group are therefore much greater.

They Offer us a Sense of Belonging and Acceptance.   Loneliness is a major problem in industrial society and group membership, which can help overcome such loneliness, is therefore often an essential feature in psychological adjustment. Interacting in a cohesive group, either at home, at work, or during leisure time, can give the individual a sense of being needed and wanted.

They Allow us to Influence Others. A group is often formed by a number of individuals in order to act as a power lobby for influencing the decision-making process. Political parties, community action groups and trade unions are all examples of groups formed to exert influence. In these instances it is a case of 'alone we are weak, together we are strong'.

Given these five important functions of groups, it is hardly surprising that humans are gregarious! However, as well as having positive outcomes, groups can also have negative effects upon the individual. The influence the presence of others has upon the individual is referred to as the 'social facilitation effect'. This refers to the finding that our level of physiological arousal increases when other people are watching us. Such arousal generally serves to increase our speed of performance, which can be either a positive or a negative state of affairs depending upon what the task is. If we are performing a simple, well learned task, then the presence of others will improve our performance, so that runners will usually achieve better times during races than in training. However, where the task is complex and we have not completely mastered it, our performance will usually deteriorate when others are watching. This deterioration is caused by what is known as 'evaluation apprehension', whereby we are worried about how other people will react to our performance.

Evaluation apprehension is obviously high during social interaction. People who are inexperienced at speaking in public, for example, tend to speak at a very fast rate due to the aforementioned increased arousal level. On the other hand, experienced public speakers will rise to the occasion when faced with a large audience, and the increased arousal level is therefore beneficial. Patients participating in SST programmes will usually have a high level of arousal caused by social anxiety initially, and will therefore find having to interact in groups doubly difficult. Their problems are summarised by Gergen and Gergen (1981) as follows:

> Being in a large group and being the focus of attention seem to create the most intense discomfort ... with strangers or members of the opposite sex posing particular difficulties ... One sample of three thousand adults reported that 'speaking

before a group' was the primary fear in life ... (and even) ...
outranked anxiety about sickness and death.

Fear of interacting in groups has been found to cause physiological reactions such as increased heart rate, perspiration and
feelings of nausea, together with impairments in intellectual performance and memory. Such fear also causes behavioural
problems in social interaction including prolonged silences,
reduced ability to break such silences, less talk time, lack of eye
contact and increased use of self-orientated gestures. Given such
findings, it is obvious that care needs to be exercised when
encouraging patients to become involved in group interaction. This
is exacerbated by the fact that patients may well have had adverse
experiences in groups in the past. An unhappy family background,
being the subject of ridicule at school or work, or being rejected in
front of others, are all experiences which will serve to increase
evaluation apprehension amongst patients. Gradually rebuilding
the confidence of patients in group situations may therefore be an
important goal of SST.

Norms

An important dimension of group dynamics relates to the norms of
particular groups. Napier and Gershenfeld (1973) define group
norms as 'ideas in the minds of members about what should and
should not be done by a specific member under certain specified
circumstances'. They further identify three main types of norms:

Formal.   Some groups will have written rules of conduct which
are available to all members. Upon taking up employment,
employees are often provided with written conditions of service
which cover expected norms of behaviour. Formal norms may also
be provided to meet specific circumstances so that, for example,
soldiers in Northern Ireland have been issued with 'yellow cards'
stating under exactly what conditions they are permitted to open
fire on suspects.

Explicitly Stated.   These are unwritten norms, but are nevertheless very strong. Thus, a new employee may be told he is expected
to wear a suit at work, and, although he does not receive such an
instruction in writing, he will come under pressure to conform to
this norm.

Informal. Every group will have a number of informal norms which are often never explicitly stated, and may only be noticed if they are violated. To a new member, these informal norms can often be difficult to decipher at first. One of the authors was once on teaching practice at a large public school and on his second morning arrived at the staff room early and sat in an inviting and comfortable chair. As the teachers arrived, he noticed one of them looking at him in a rather agitated fashion before leaving the room. One of his colleagues then approached with the information that this chair was 'Mr. X's'. Upon enquiring further, it was discovered that, in fact, each teacher had his 'own' chair in the staff room. Although this was an unofficial and unspoken arrangement, it was also an important informal norm. The author then learned to occupy one of the chairs reserved for student teachers!

Norms are very useful in that 'they increase the regularity and predictability of social behaviour ... (prevent) conflict, stabilize relationships and moderate the use of power' (Keisler 1978). Thus, norms facilitate the interaction process in groups since they provide parameters about which behaviours are, or are not, acceptable. Breaking or deviating from these accepted norms will usually result in sanctions of some form being taken against the 'offender', including in extreme cases being expelled from the group. However, not all deviants will necessarily be rejected by a group. Someone who has been a valuable member of a group in the past and made valuable contributions therein, will have built up 'idiosyncrasy credits' allowing him a certain leeway to deviate from the expected norms. Such individuals will also be most influential in changing the norms of a group (Shaw, 1981).

Apart from this exception, people who do not adhere to group norms will experience problems. When someone deviates in a group, that person may receive a lot of communications from other group members initially, in an attempt to persuade them to conform. If the deviance persists, however, they will be thrown out (either literally or metaphorically!) of the group. It is therefore important for patients to be aware of the norms of particular groups, and to realise the implications of breaking them. In general, many patients are rejected by others in society because they behave in an abnormal fashion.

Group Factors

A number of factors should be taken into consideration when

covering the topic of participating in groups, and encouraging patients to engage in such participation. These include:

Size.   It is obviously easier to contribute in a group, comprising a total of three members, than a group of 30. However, it is easier to remain anonymous in a larger group, whereas in a small group each member is under pressure to contribute. As a group becomes larger, one person in the group will tend to do more talking (Gulley 1968). This is because leadership, and in particular the necessity for control, becomes more important as group size increases. During SST it is useful to concentrate on small group involvement where groups should not exceed six members. Ideally, patients should be encouraged to participate in dyads initially when learning the main social skills. Once a level of confidence has been built up, the group size should be gradually increased to the maximum group size wherein the patient would be expected to contribute actively.

Degree of Participation.   Patients may contribute to groups without a great deal of difficulty if they are not the specific focus of attention. A classic example of this would be participating in a church service, where each person is really acting individually although part of an overall group, and no member of the congregation really plays a central role. Where the patient is to be the focus of attention for at least some of the time as part of an interacting group, the problems become greater, since evaluation apprehension is prevalent. In SST it can be useful to acclimatise patients to groups by allowing them initially to play a passive role, and gradually getting them more involved.

Control.   The feeling of being in control, or part of the system of control, is important for group members. When people feel that they have no control over a situation or event, their unhappiness and anxiety levels tend to increase. For example, it has been found that subjects in an experiment perceived a lift to be less crowded and larger than it actually was if they were standing beside, as opposed to away from, the control panel. In terms of social interaction, an improvement in social ability following SST results in an increased level of personal confidence and a correspondingly greater feeling of being 'in control' in group situations. If a group approach to SST is adopted it is important to involve patients actively at every stage of the programme. This can be achieved by distributing tasks individually to patients, and then allowing patients to make their own contributions to the overall group. For instance, if a video-tape is being shown in which nonverbal communication is to be analysed, each patient could be given the task of making some notes about one particular aspect (e.g. posture, gestures) and would then feed these comments back into an overall discussion about the tape. This technique can help to give patients some degree of control over the training programme, and thereby increase their enjoyment of the exercise itself.

Physical Environment. Interaction within groups can be encouraged by manipulating the physical environment. It has been found that in housing estates people tend to become friends with those who live either beside or directly opposite one another, because they are more likely to come into direct contact. In the same way, the furniture in a room can be arranged so that people are more likely to interact by, for example, moving chairs together in small circles as opposed to having them spaced out along the walls of a room. (Such an approach has been successfully employed in several studies of old people's institutions with marked increases in interaction between residents.) The implications for running SST programmes are fairly obvious.

Risk. In any group discussion an individual who makes a contribution is always taking some degree of risk, in that he may be scorned or ridiculed by other group members. As discussed in Chapter 7, different public situations will have differing degrees of risk. Care must be taken not to expose patients too early to high risk situations (such as discos or dances) where there is a possibility of being rejected by others. The degree of risk in groups is reduced where:

(1) A leader is present to control interaction and protect group members
(2) The individual can, if desired, remain anonymous at times within the group
(3) There is a practical task being carried out by each individual, but no group evaluation of each member's efforts
(4) It is possible to interact with one group member at a time without other members listening.

These points should be borne in mind when designing homework tasks for patients. Situations of low risk include courses or classes at colleges and leisure centres, such as keep fit, swimming or car maintenance. Although the focus of such activity is practical, friendships quite often develop between group members. Depending upon the interests of patients, they might also join a rambling or a jogging/running club.

Overview

The four elements of social interaction covered in this chapter are all important areas of study for nurses to consider during SST. The central skills of asking questions and giving explanations will be of relevance to all patients. The ability to use questioning techniques skilfully can improve both the confidence and performance levels of patients. Questions serve both to express interest in others and take the pressure off the patient. Similarly, explaining is a skill that is used frequently during social encounters to convey information to others. The ability to explain personal experiences, opinions or feelings in a coherent and cogent fashion will contribute significantly to inter-personal competence.

For some patients, learning how to be assertive will be an important feature of SST. The nurse needs to ascertain in exactly what situations patients experience difficulty in being assertive, and then concentrate on overcoming these problems. Finally, having to interact in the presence of a number of other people will cause specific difficulties for many patients. For most of us, the presence of others will increase our levels of arousal, but for those who have high levels of social anxiety initially, this increased arousal can be severely dysfunctional.

9 RESPONDING SKILLS

Both the effectiveness and maintenance of inter-personal communication depend greatly on the response one receives from the person with whom one is interacting. Certain sections of the psychiatrically ill population have difficulty responding appropriately when interacting, and as a result communication is often seen as unrewarding with resultant termination of conversation. The inability to respond appropriately socially not only handicaps the patient in establishing new acquaintances but often also affects existing relationships.

In this chapter the 'responding' skills used while interacting will be discussed. Four skill areas in this category are included. Firstly, listening, which enables one both to understand and to communicate interest in and feelings about what the other is saying. Secondly, skills used to respond to feeling enabling one to achieve a deeper, fuller appreciation of the other as an individual. Thirdly, reflecting skills, used to encourage a person to continue talking on a particular topic and expand upon what they have already said. The final section of the chapter will examine skills of rewardingness which help to determine, by means of reinforcement, the nature and duration of interaction.

Listening

Research indicates that many people are poor listeners. Listening skill is not a natural ability but must be worked at and developed over a period of time. Taking cognisance of this, one can appreciate more fully how psychiatrically ill patients experience particular difficulty with this aspect of interaction. Either as a precursor or as a consequence of the illness, psychiatric patients frequently have problems in receiving and assimilating information during communication. Recognition must be taken of this during the rehabilitatory phase. In order to function appropriately in a social setting (e.g. shopping, banking, ordering, enquiring, socialising), discharged patients need to be taught how to listen effectively.

Defining the term 'listening' can be problematic since opinions differ as to what is entailed. Some researchers, for example, feel it involves the perception of any sounds. This includes not only the spoken word but also paralanguage (as discussed in Chapter 7), which helps determine the precise meaning of what is said. Others believe listening to include only the spoken word or the language part of the communication. In so doing attention is given to what is actually being said without taking cognisance of how it is said. A third school of thought believes listening to encompass both the perception of speech and other stimuli. In addition to language and paralanguage, such exponents feel that listening entails also the nonvocal aspects of interaction, including physical appearance, body movements, facial expression etc. Finally, certain exponents emphasise the perceptual processing of data in listening. Here, while an array of stimuli bombard the listener from many different sources and through several sensory organs, an effective listener via a process of selective perception (see Chapter 4; Figure 4.6) attends only to that which enables him to receive and assimilate the speaker's message and in turn respond accordingly. Patients suffering from schizophrenia occasionally have difficulty in both receiving and assimilating the speaker's message. This may be typically seen where they cannot attend selectively, being over-inclusive in their perception.

The definition adopted in this text is that suggested by Smith (1986) which takes into account the above four schools of thought. Smith defined listening as 'an active process that involves all sounds the communication participants produce, intentional or unintentional, that they perceive and which may be influenced by various non-auditory factors associated with the context'.

Types of Listening

As there are different definitions of listening, so too are there different types. The types 'active' or 'passive' listening are perhaps misleading in that they may have different meanings for different people. A commonly held view, for example, is that passive listening merely involves one effortlessly receiving messages from another. This view tends to place a heavy burden of responsibility upon the source suggesting that the speaker is the one who controls or determines the communication. It tends to accord the listener no more than a minor or insignificant role. In the strictest sense of the word, however, passive listening as defined by Hargie

et al (1981) emphasises the cognitive process of assimilating information. In passive listening (sometimes referred to as covert) the
receiver displays no outward signs or behaviour to indicate that
listening is taking place. Bearing in mind the above definition,
passive listening is by no means an effortless process. It demands
active participation on the part of the listener, as he concentrates
on searching for meaning and understanding in the message being
conveyed. The term passive listening is then perhaps a misnomer
as the receiver needs to select actively what he wishes to attend to
and then process and assimilate the information chosen.

In active or overt listening the receiver, in addition to assimilating the information selected, displays certain behaviours which
indicate that he is paying attention to the speaker. In most
instances this type of listening is preferable since it affords the
speaker feedback on what is being said. Such feedback not only
shows that listening has taken place but also may encourage the
speaker to continue. In terms of social skills it is active listening
that is utilised. The verbal and nonverbal aspects of behaviour
which convey the impression of active listening will be examined
later in this section.

When discussing the types of listening, cognisance must be
taken of the context in which it is used. If a patient, for example,
during a social occasion were to sit and listen passively to what is
going on, their apparent lack of interest or inattentiveness would
quickly result in their exclusion from the interaction. When
improving a patient's listening skills, therefore, attention must not
only be given to the receiving and assimilating of information but
also the patient's ability to respond appropriately while listening.

Effective Listening

Having differentiated between active and passive listening and
identified the use of the former in SST, it is now necessary to
examine more closely those responses that are associated wih
effective listening. The definition of listening given earlier in this
section emphasises the importance of attending to both the
speaker's verbal and nonverbal cues. Similarly, the speaker while
transmitting a message 'listens' for the receiver's verbal and nonverbal responses. Obtaining such feedback, as suggested by
Rosenfeld and Hancks (1980), is an integral part of the communication process. When a person is speaking, for example, they need
feedback on how their listeners are responding, so that they can

modify their remarks accordingly. They need to know whether their listeners understand, believe, are surprised or bored, agree or disagree, are pleased or annoyed. This information is obtained from 'signals' from the listener. An early head-nod indicates understanding, a raised eyebrow signals surprise, and so on.

While verbal responses are important indicators of effective listening, the receiver's nonverbal behaviour (e.g. paralanguage, body language) may either help to accentuate listening or conversely highlight inattentiveness or lack of interest. Certain psychiatric patients may occasionally present with mismatched verbal and nonverbal behaviour while listening, resulting in ambiguous and confusing feedback for the speaker. Patients, for example, who experience incongruity of mood, may appear verbally to say one thing and nonverbally convey something else. In effective listening, therefore, recognition should be given to both the receiver's verbal and nonverbal responses and the way in which they are synchronised.

When considering the elements of effective listening, recognition should be given to the following. Firstly, anyone who wishes to be an effective listener must, as suggested by Smith (1986):

> be willing to expend the effort to permit others to express their feelings and ideas. To do this one must be willing to give something of oneself. This requires that the person must first be *receptive*. Receptiveness is a deliberate action consciously performed with the intention of relating in some way to the other.

By creating a climate that is accepting and supportive, the listener conveys his or her concern and respect, encouraging the speaker to confide and ventilate. As the person talks the listener should encourage them to continue by acknowledging them verbally. This might be achieved through what Spence (1980) termed as attention feedback. This involves small, minimal response cues which signal attention and understanding and also help reinforce the speaker's message. Appropriate comments such as 'yes', 'I see', 'ah ha' and 'hmmm' may help add to the listener's receptiveness. Such verbal reinforcers, however, must be used appropriately because their misuse (e.g. the same one used too often, excessive use of superlatives to the extent they are rendered meaningless) could result in their having little or even a contrary effect on the speaker. Rosenshine (1971), for example, points out that it is simple to administer positive reinforcers without much thought, but in order to demonstrate genuine listening some reasons have to be given for the use of the reinforcers.

A second criterion for effective listening is one's ability to pay attention to what is said. In so doing one should not be pre-occupied with oneself but make a conscious effort to exhibit active signs of attentiveness. This can be achieved in a variety of ways, both verbally and nonverbally and include:

(1) Verbal following, as described by Hargie et al (1981), where the listener, by matching his verbal comments closely to the responses of the speaker, conveys attentiveness and interest

(2) Attentive posturing, e.g. open stance, leaning towards speaker, sideways tilt of head

(3) Mirroring facial expressions of the speaker in order to reflect and express sympathy with the emotional message being conveyed

(4) Head movements used at the appropriate time, to indicate willingness to listen and agreement with what is being said

(5) Paralanguage (as described earlier) which can indicate the listener's enthusiasm for the message being emitted (e.g. appropriate tone of voice, loudness and so on).

A third important aspect in effective listening is one's ability to use silence appropriately. In silence people can express many feelings ranging from love and concern through to hostility and resent-ment. Too frequently patients, perhaps due to social anxiety or lack of self-confidence, find it difficult to use silence properly. As a consequence they interrupt the speaker too frequently or con-versely their silence, accompanied by other negative nonverbal cues, may be construed as lack of interest in what is being said. In using silence effectively, the listener should not only remain quiet but must also intimate through appropriate nonverbal behaviour that such silence is out of respect and concern for the speaker. Many of the nonverbal behaviours that would accompany silence to indicate interest and concern have already been mentioned, (e.g. attentive posture, head movements). Other social skills ele-ments that would accentuate the use of silence include:

(1) Direct eye contact, which helps inform the speaker of the listener's attentiveness and interest, assists also in conveying

warmth, and sincerity

(2) By smiling appropriately, one can indicate to the speaker without talking, friendliness, feelings about conversational topic and ability to understand the message

(3) Touch and physical contact are powerful ways of communicating emotions and comfort and as stated by Blondis and Jackson (1977) 'can be even more meaningful if used without words'.

To use silence effectively it is essential for the listener to be patient. Listening requires more patience than perhaps any other human activity. Too frequently people, because of their impatience to talk, fail to listen properly to the speaker. This is typically seen in the people who are so preoccupied with what they are going to say that they fail to listen to the other's point of view. Consequently their verbal and nonverbal cues create an impression of inattentiveness and lack of interest.

A fourth criterion for effective listening is ensuring that our actions, as listeners, are clear and unambiguous so that they do not mislead the speaker. Avoiding ambiguity will entail asking pertinent probing questions and seeking clarification when the message is not fully understood. Probing questions are a direct form of listening, wherein one follows up the responses of the speaker by asking related questions. Such questions are designed to encourage the speaker to expand upon initial responses. They can be used where the listener is unsure of the content or meaning of the message and seeks to elicit a clearer understanding of what the speaker is saying. Because of irregularities in perceiving and thinking and as a result of the side effects of drugs, patients often have difficulty fully comprehending and interpreting messages. By using clarification probes such as 'What exactly do you mean?' or 'Are you saying that ...?' patients can obtain a greater appreciation of the speaker's meaning.

Important also in effective listening is the minimising or removal of distractions while attending. As stated earlier, the speaker while transmitting a message listens for the receiver's verbal and nonverbal responses. If the receiver engages in distracting behaviour such as fidgeting, doodling, acknowledging other people or things in the immediate surroundings, it quickly becomes apparent that they are not fully committed to the conversation nor interested in what is being said. Listeners, to be effective, must refrain from such activities. This may entail stopping and putting aside what one is doing (e.g. work, eating) so attention can be given fully to the speaker. Distractions, however, may not be under the listener's control but may arise from the environment within which the interaction takes place. The listener who is truly concerned about providing full attention will seek to overcome distractions from extraneous stimuli, should they be sounds, sights or even smells. This might include the removal to a more suitable environment or steps being taken to minimise the existing distractions (e.g. turning off machinery, closing a door, or requesting others to be quiet). Such actions would indicate to the speaker the listener's willingness to attend fully to the message being conveyed.

A sixth criterion for effective listening is the ability to grasp the full meaning of the speaker's message so seeking agreement on what is being said. Although focusing can be useful in helping the speaker to expand on a topic of importance and keep the communication process goal-directed, the listener should search to find the broader meaning rather than concentrating on certain words and sentences. By focusing too specifically on isolated facts, certain meanings can be deduced out of context and distort the overall message conveyed. A good listener, therefore, must not attend too closely to particular aspects to the detriment of others, but should seek to identify the overall theme of the speaker's communication.

Finally, an effective listener in order not to prejudge a situation must delay evaluating listening until he is sure that he understands fully the other person's position. This may be achieved in several ways, including:

(1) By paraphrasing the listener summarises, in his own words, the essential meaning of the speaker's message. This not only helps establish that the listener understands the full meaning of the message, but also encourages the speaker to continue talking and illustrates that accurate listening has taken place.
(2) By summarising, the listener brings together the main thoughts, ideas, facts and feelings at the end of or during a conversation. Such an exercise, as suggested by Brammer (1979): 'Helps to finish a conversation on a natural note, to clarify and focus a series of scattered ideas, and clear the way for new ideas. It has the effect of reassurance. The patient knows that you have understood all of what has been said'.

Such exercises enable the listener to gain a fuller understanding of what has been said. Only once this has been achieved can evaluation of the message take place.

The above criteria are associated with attentiveness. Although listening can occur without displaying such overt signs, it is socially preferable, for various reasons, to demonstrate that listening is taking place.

Obstacles to Effective Listening

In order accurately to receive and assimilate the messages of others one must first be aware of those obstacles that could militate against effective listening. Such obstacles, for purposes of clarity, can be loosely classified into three groups, namely: obstacles emanating from the speaker, the listener and other circumstances (see Figure 9.1).

Figure 9.1: Obstacles to Effective Listening

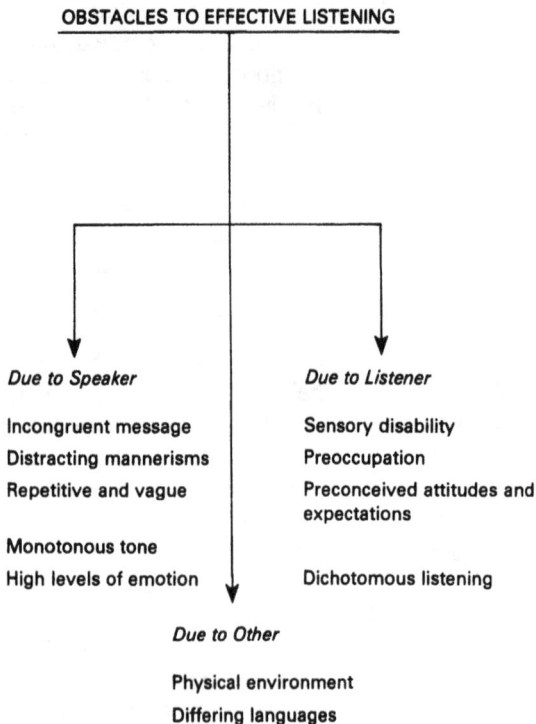

OBSTACLES TO EFFECTIVE LISTENING

Due to Speaker

Incongruent message
Distracting mannerisms
Repetitive and vague

Monotonous tone
High levels of emotion

Due to Listener

Sensory disability
Preoccupation
Preconceived attitudes and
expectations

Dichotomous listening

Due to Other

Physical environment
Differing languages

Speaker Obstacles. When the speaker's verbal and nonverbal messages are complementary (i.e. convey similar meaning) the communication is termed congruent. If, however, the person verbally says one thing and nonverbally implies something else, the message is termed incongruent and can be problematic for the listener.

(1) Congruent communication:
    Verbal message: 'I'm pleased to see you'
    Nonverbal message: Voice sounds warm, continuous eye contact, smiling.
(2) Incongruent communication:
    Verbal message: 'I'm, pleased to see you'
    Nonverbal message: Voice sounds cold and distant, avoids eye contact, neutral facial expression.

Incongruent or double-level messages produce a dilemma for the listener because they do not know which message to respond to, verbal or nonverbal. Since they cannot respond to both, they are likely to feel frustrated, angry, or confused.

The speaker may also, because of certain distracting mannerisms, detract from the message conveyed. Anomalies, including the presence of a stutter or lisp, or perhaps the use of excessive gesticulation, can redirect the listener's attention away from the actual communication. Repetitiveness or lengthy and irrelevant dialogue presented in a monotonous fashion can lead to the listener 'turning off'. This may be seen where the subject of conversation is boring and where the speaker is perhaps vague and unsure of the topic. Lastly, the speaker by being in a highly charged emotional state can distract the listener from attending fully to the verbal message. A person who is too emotional often becomes illogical in his argument and fails to listen to the other's point of view. It is advisable, in such a situation, for the listener to sustain (i.e. encourage to ventilate) the interaction allowing the emotion to subside. Such emotion can also give rise to anxiety within the listener, interfering with his ability to listen effectively.

Listener Obstacles. In some instances the speaker's message is clear and unambiguous, but listening is ineffective due to anomalies in receiving. The listener may be inattentive for some reason, and may not be giving his full attention to what is being said. Preoccupation for example, with a forthcoming important appointment, a recently held social function, or even one's self-image can militate against effective listening. Concern about the impression one is creating may result in little attention being paid to the speaker's message.

The listener's previous experience, attitudes, values and feelings can also be an obstacle to effective and objective listening. The listener's attitudes, for example, generate expectations which in turn influence that to which he will attend. In so doing he tends to interpret the speaker's cues in such a way as to maintain consistency with his own beliefs. Finally, dichotomous listening, which occurs when an individual attempts to assimilate information simultaneously from two different sources, may interfere with the ability of the listener to attend effectively, since messages may be either received inaccurately or not received at all.

Other Obstacles.   Extraneous distractions, as described earlier (i.e. machinery, lack of privacy), which are outside the control of the speaker and listener can distort both the emission and reception of the message. In attempting to overcome noise, for example, the speaker may raise his voice and exaggerate movements to compensate. In so doing the true meaning of the communication may be weakened. Likewise, the listener may be unable to hear all of the message or may perhaps be distracted by other stimuli. Either way, obstacles in the physical environment can militate against both emission of the message and effective listening. Finally, where the speaker and listener do not share the same language and/or nonverbal conventions, listening is inevitably impoverished. The degree of impoverishment will vary depending on the languages concerned, some being closer and more similar than others. Partial obstacles may also be set up when the speaker and the listener both use the same language but with different dialects.

In conclusion, listening is more than merely a simple process of hearing. It demands both conscious and committed effort on the part of the receiver with a knowledge of not only the necessary complimentary skills but also the obstacles that might militate against effective listening.

Empathy

Empathy is a characteristic that is difficult to describe, but is relatively easy for people to perceive in an effective communicator. The term represents something fundamental in a person's manner and is of importance in creating an environment that is both non-threatening and accepting. The lack or absence of empathetic ability in many psychiatric patients often creates an interactional barrier, whereby their 'cold' and 'removed' manner is construed as unfriendliness and unacceptance. Much of the problem stems from emotional disturbances. Depression, elation, shallowing or incongruity of mood can affect the patient's perceptions and consequently their responses. The inability to perceive accurately and respond appropriately often hinders the psychiatric patient from empathising effectively. This undoubtedly can inhibit the behaviour of others with whom the patient is interacting and as a result sustained communication may be avoided. Such a situation can often give rise to a cyclic effect involving both the patient and the person with whom he is communicating (see Figure 9.2).

Schafer (1959) defined empathy as: 'An experience which takes place between two or more individuals. It is basically the ability to

Figure 9.2: Relationship between Behaviour and Emotions in Empathy

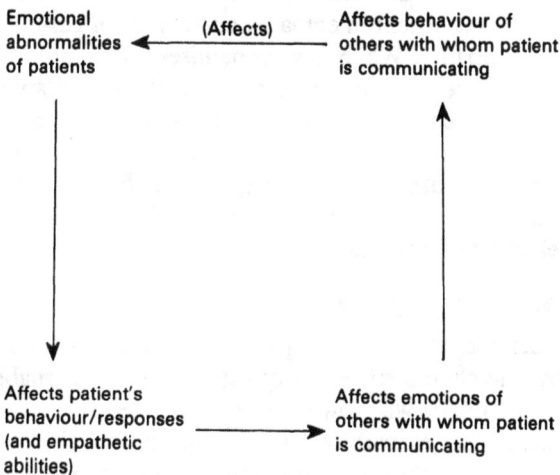

enter into, or share in and comprehend the momentary psycho-logical state of another individual.'

This theme is also found in the definition given by Kalisch (1973) who defines empathy as 'the ability to enter into the life of another person, to accurately perceive his current feelings and meanings'. These definitions emphasise the ability to understand the meaning and relevance of the thoughts and feelings of the individual concerned. In addition, French (1983) describes this ability to appreciate another person's thoughts and feelings from his point of view, as 'advanced empathy'. 'Primary empathy', he suggests, is synonymous with active listening (as already described in this chapter) which shows that the listener has received and understood the speaker's point of view. Joyce Travelbee (1971), in agreeing with Schafer's definition, emphasises also the need to stand apart from the object of one's empathy. This apart-ness in empathy, she states, 'does not imply a cold objectivity, rather it implies a sense of sharing while being detached from the object of one's empathy'. This objectiveness of empathy and the subjective-ness of sympathy is, at times, unclear.

Empathy and Sympathy

Sympathy, in many ways, can be seen as a progression from the empathetic process. Where empathy is concerned with the ability to perceive accurately another's current feelings and meanings, sympathy in addition wishes to alleviate the other's distress.

As suggested by Travelbee (1971), this desire to alleviate the other's distress is absent in empathy and is a distinguishing charac-teristic of sympathy. When one empathises one is not affected by that which concerns another, and although understanding what another is experiencing there is no desire to do anything to aid the distress. Conversely, sympathetic persons are concerned and wish to assist, not because it is their assigned role, but because they are motivated by compassion. Compassion underlies and is a funda-mental element of sympathy.

Characteristics of Empathy

Having defined the term empathy and differentiated it from sympathy, the characteristics or qualities that would enable one to be more empathetic will now be examined.

The ability to empathise varies with the speaker, time and listener. Undoubtedly a general interest in people, basic knowledge of human behaviour and cultural customs, and a warm, flexible personality will encourage empathy. Other characteristics that would enable one to be more empathetic include:

(1) Verbal and nonverbal behaviour should be focused on by the listener.
(2) By being able to use a variety of words, phrases and statements that are expressive of emotion, the listener should formulate responses of empathy in a language and manner that is most easily understood by the speaker.
(3) The tone of the listener's response should be similar to that of the speaker and convey, verbally and nonverbally, warmth and spontaneity.
(4) In addition to concentrating on what is being expressed, the listener should also be aware of what is not being expressed. This will entail listening with a 'third ear', becoming involved in the other and abandoning self-consciousness.
(5) The listener must be able to interpret correctly, without distortion, the speaker's responses, and use them as a guide in developing future responses. By using responses tactfully, the listener can move the interview in the direction of the speaker's feelings and concerns.
(6) The listener must be able to abstract the core or essential meaning of the speaker's feelings and concerns and discuss them in acceptable terms.
(7) Finally, the listener in order to empathise effectively must be able to cope with egocentricity, anxiety, fears or other feelings or stresses that might interfere with listening to and feeling with another.

In addition to the above, Beckmann-Murray and Wilson-Huelskoetter (1983) identified specific verbal and nonverbal behaviours that convey high levels of empathy. One must, they suggest, face the person and maintain eye contact, adopt an open relaxed posture, lean towards the other and use verbal and non-verbal communication so that the person experiences a feeling of being understood. In empathising, they continued, one should reflect the person's feelings frequently and tentatively for correction, clarification, elaboration and validation, and remain open to the response. A person who feels free to correct the other moves onto a higher level of self-understanding. Empathising requires one also to focus on feelings rather than content, referring only to the content when the feelings have been determined. Lastly, one must avoid vague generalities while attempting to convey empathy. When reflecting and paraphrasing it is essential to use precise words and statements to describe and clarify accurately the other's feelings.

Barriers to Empathy

The ability to perceive accurately another's current feelings and meanings depends greatly upon the similarities of experience between the two persons involved. It can be difficult for the listener to fully appreciate another's point of view if he himself has not experienced what the speaker is talking about. This area has received much attention in recent years. For example, research by Halpern and Lesser (1960) conclude that: 'A person's ability to empathise with similar people lies strictly with the boundaries of their similarity and disappears in personality areas in which they differ.'

Lack of similarity or differences, therefore, between the speaker and listener can create barriers to the empathetic process. Differences, for example, in sex, age, religion, socio-economic status, education and culture can block the development of empathetic understanding. Because everyone is individually unique, no one can completely understand another person. However, the wider a person's background and the more varied their experiences, the greater will be their potential for understanding people. The potential to empathise effectively can be enhanced in an individual, through such exercises as role-playing and relevant background reading. These exercises are designed so as to enhance appreciation and understanding of others' position and circumstances (see Chapter 10).

In addition to similarity, another barrier to the development of empathy may be the lack of desire to share in and comprehend the momentary psychological state of another individual. Experience of and insight into another's circumstances is of little use in the development of empathy if the desire or intent to understand is lacking. Alternatively, the wish to empathise could be present but the motives for doing so could be for manipulation or exploitation as opposed to helping the person.

In conclusion, in order to empathise effectively cognisance must be taken of the similarities and differences between individuals and the roles they play in the development of empathy. Recognition must also be given to the extent to which, and reasons why, one wishes to empathise with another.

Reflecting

The skill of reflecting, although evolved from and central to the counselling process, is also an important feature of effective communication in many everyday interactions. Effective reflecting requires the listener to be sensitive, perceptive and concise in his interpretation of the speaker's message, and consequently such demands often result in the skill being used inappropriately and inaccurately. The integrated nature of reflection makes it one of the most difficult social skills to master. It must be appreciated, therefore, that additional difficulties, as found in certain psychiatric conditions (e.g. inability to attend closely to and interpret the speaker's message) can further impede one from using the skill effectively.

Reflection, as suggested by Hargie et al (1981), is the process of mirroring back in the interviewer's own words, 'the essence of the interviewee's previous statement'. As there are different types of information conveyed during interaction so too are there different types of reflection. One type of information is primarily factual or cognitive concerning ideas, thoughts, places, events, objects and the like. The second type is essentially concerned with the feeling or affective aspect of the message and includes emotions such as anger, fear, anxiety, confusion, joy, elation and so on. While exponents such as Becvar (1974), Horan (1979) and French (1983) include both reflection of feeling and content in their definitions, others including Ivey and Authier (1978), Athos and Gabarro (1978) and Hargie et al (1981) consider there to be different types of reflection for the two different types of information, namely:

(1) Reflection of content — more commonly referred to as paraphrasing
(2) Reflection of feeling.

In identifying the two different types of reflection, however, it is generally recognised that they share a number of salient characteristics. Looking at each as distinct from the other is therefore difficult since much overlapping can occur. This vagueness in differentiation is recognised by Ivey and Authier (1978) who state: 'Just as reflection of feeling entails some reiteration of content so paraphrasing entails some recognition of feelings. The primary distinction is emphasis.'

Reflection of Feeling

The term reflection of feeling, as suggested by Ivey and Authier (1978), can be described as the 'selective attention to the feeling or emotional aspects of the speaker's message.' This definition, however, fails to emphasise the importance of feedback in the reflective process. Hargie et al (1981) in their definition describe the term as: 'The process of feeding back to the interviewee in the interviewer's own words, the essence of the interviewee's previous statement, the emphasis being upon feelings expressed rather than cognitive content.' The purpose of reflecting feelings is to focus on feelings rather than the content of the message. The feeling component may be expressed in several ways and can at times be difficult to determine. Firstly, feelings may be expressed explicitly, whereby certain words clearly highlight the feelings of the person. Secondly, feelings may be implicitly expressed where an emotional message is contained within the statement facts. The restaurant customer, for example, who has been waiting a long time for service says, bitingly, 'Do you think you could manage some service over here, please.' Finally, the feeling component of the message may be inferred, whereby the manner in which the verbal content is delivered (i.e. nonverbal and paralinguistics) conveys the person's inner feelings. The skilful use of this technique, therefore, depends greatly on the listener's ability to identify feelings from the speaker's verbal and nonverbal behaviours.

Steps in reflection of feeling have been provided by Cormier and Cormier (1979), Ivey and Authier (1978) and Stuart and Sundeen (1983) which include:

(1) Recall and restate the speaker's message covertly
(2) Determine what feelings are being expressed by identifying the affect words used or the nonverbal cues
(3) Translate the speaker's feelings into your own words at about the same level of intensity
(4) Verbally reflect the speaker's feelings in statement form, using

in addition certain paraphrased elements of the speaker's past statement

(5) Judge by the reaction of the speaker whether the reflection was correct or not.

Sometimes even inaccurate reflections can be facilitative because the speaker may correct the listener and state his feelings more clearly.

Functions of Reflection of Feeling. Reflecting feelings has several functions, and although in many instances these are similar to the functions of paraphrasing, they differ in certain areas. Firstly, by reflecting feeling accurately the listener demonstrates not only attention and interest in the speaker but also attaches importance and respect to the message conveyed. Secondly, by mirroring back the essence of the speaker's feelings contained in the message, the listener is able to check the accuracy of their own understanding. If the reflection is accurate the speaker will continue, if it is not he can correct the misinterpretation. Thirdly, reflection of feeling enables the speaker to realise that the listener is aware of the emotions emitted. This, in turn, leads to a more trusting and empathetic relationship. If one, for example, realises that the other is making an effort to understand what is being said, then one is more likely to continue to divulge more information. Fourthly, the technique of reflection can encourage the speaker to explore and express his feelings (both positive and negative) about certain situations. In so doing they can be made to realise that feelings can have an important causal influence upon their actions. Finally, by reflecting feelings one indicates to the speaker that it is acceptable for them both to have and to express such feelings in that situation. The feelings conveyed during interaction are all too often ignored, suppressed and in some societies even frowned upon. Any attempts to demonstrate feelings explicitly may cause embarrassment, consequently resulting in the termination of communication. Identification and acceptance of one's feelings, therefore, is of paramount importance in the reflective process. Failure to do so will result in only superficial conversation being reached.

Incorrect Use of Reflection of Feeling. Although reflection of feeling is a very useful technique, it is often difficult to master effectively. As a result the process is frequently used incorrectly.

Stuart and Sundeen (1983), for example, identified several difficulties or errors in reflecting feeling accurately:

(1) Stereotyping one's responses. Continually beginning reflections in the same monotonous way (such as 'you feel') may give the impression of an automatic, thoughtless response which can have a detrimental effect on the interaction.
(2) Reflecting back everything that is said. This can provoke feelings of irritation, anger and frustration in the speaker, and may give the appearance of insincerity and superficiality on the part of the listener.
(3) Infrequent reflection of feeling. Conversely the listener may reflect too infrequently, either because they dislike interrupting the speaker or because of inappropriate timing. Either way it is difficult to 'capture' a feeling after it has passed.
(4) Inappropriate use of language. The language used can be inappropriate to the cultural experience and educational level of the speaker; effective language is that which is natural to the listener and readily understood by the speaker.
(5) Inappropriate depth of feeling. The listener fails to reflect appropriately by either being too superficial in assessment of the speaker's feelings or conversely being too deep.

In addition to the above Hargie et al (1981) highlight the problems of reflecting feelings inaccurately. Inaccurate reflecting, as stated earlier, can be useful where the speaker may correct the listener and state his feelings more clearly. Persistent inaccurate reflecting, however, may indicate to the speaker that the listener is not on the same 'wavelength' and fails to grasp what is being said. Finally, Athos and Gabarro (1978), elaborating on inappropriate depth of feeling (as previously identified by Stuart and Sundeen), describe the difficulties associated with over- and under-reaching the speaker's feelings. Over-reaching or over-rating the depth of feeling, they suggest, will result in the speaker feeling misunderstood and questioning the other's capacity to grasp the affective component of the message. Going too far, they add, can be construed as the listener taking liberties, making up their own meanings from what the speaker has said. Conversely, by under-reaching or under-rating the depth of feeling, no real insight is gained of the speaker's innermost feelings, resulting in the situation being explored staying at a superficial level. This frequently occurs when the listener responds to the content rather than the feeling component of the message.

Reflection of Content

Reflection of content, more commonly referred to as paraphrasing, as suggested by Monti et al (1982), simply requires the listener to summarise what the speaker has said. The emphasis, as stated earlier, is on the cognitive or factual components of the message rather than affect. Hargie et al (1981) suggest that there are three important elements inherent in the definition of paraphrasing. Firstly, the paraphrase should be summarised in the listener's own words. This should not be confused with the technique of echoing whereby one is simply concerned with repeating what has just been said. Paraphrasing, in addition, entails the listener using their own words and phrases to encapsulate the essence of what is being communicated. Secondly, the paraphrase should contain the essential components of the previous statement. This may be rather difficult at times since the central components of the message may be embedded in para — or irrelevant — dialogue. Lastly, paraphrasing is primarily concerned with reflecting the factual information received. Although it largely ignores feelings expressed, cognisance may be unwittingly taken of both components of the message.

Like the technique of reflecting feelings there are, as suggested by Cormier and Cormier (1979) and Stuart and Sundeen (1983), certain steps in effective paraphrasing including:

(1) Attend to and recall the speaker's factual message covertly
(2) Identify the core or essential factual components of the message
(3) Translate and verbalise the factual component of the message in your own words
(4) Judge by the reaction of the speaker whether the paraphrase was correct or not.

Functions of Paraphrasing

Certain functions of paraphrasing have already been mentioned in the section on reflecting feelings, but their importance nevertheless warrants their inclusion again. Firstly, by paraphrasing the factual content of a message accurately the listener conveys their interest and concern to the speaker, and that they are paying full attention to what is being said. Secondly, by summarising in their own words the essence of the message content, the listener can check the accuracy of their understanding and at the same time imprint on their memory what has been said. Doing so helps clarify the ideas that the speaker is expressing and validates the listener's understanding of the speaker's meaning. Thirdly, it affords feedback for the speaker, enabling them to see that the other is on the same 'wavelength'. Fourthly, paraphrasing helps guide and encourage the speaker to continue talking, and to talk at greater depth. By creating an aura of acceptance through outwardly displaying interest, concern and understanding the speaker is encouraged to ventilate further. Fifthly, by mirroring back the essence of the speaker's factual message the listener can tie a number of comments together and highlight issues by stating them more concisely. Finally, paraphrasing accurately enables the speaker to focus on particular aspects of the message more closely. This allows them to expand on certain salient issues and keeps the communication process goal-directed. Intense focusing, however, may be rather anxiety-producing and consequently detrimental to the relationship. Effectively used, it can help the speaker become more specific, move from vagueness to clarity, and focus on reality.

The technique of paraphrasing can be of immense value particularly with certain types of psychiatric patient who, because of being circumstantial in conversation, tend to be constantly vague and superficial.

In conclusion the art of reflecting accurately requires great skill on the part of the listener. Although perhaps one of the most difficult social skills to master, research evidence indicates that performance of this skill can be improved considerably by means of training programmes (Ivey et al, 1968; Goldberg, 1971).

Skills of Rewardingness

Being social creatures, we like the company of other people. During social encounters we are continually rewarding and reinforcing each other by the attention we give and receive. Inherent in the skills already discussed in this chapter is the importance of rewarding or reinforcing the other's behaviour. When actively listening to a person, for example, by displaying certain behaviours (e.g. head nodding, forward leaning posture) one indicates

attention and interest and in so doing encourages the other to continue interacting. Unfortunately, one of the most common characteristics of socially unskilled psychiatric patients is their low level
of rewardingness. This is particularly the case in chronic schizophrenia where patients have been described by Longabaugh et al
(1966) as being 'socially bankrupt'. The inability to provide social
reward or reinforcement, both verbally and nonverbally, frequently results in the cessation of communication. The role of
reward by means of reinforcement is therefore an integral process
in social skills sequences and so necessitates closer examination.

In order to appreciate fully the significance of reinforcement in
SST it is perhaps pertinent to review briefly the theoretical background. Although greatly debated by many theorists, the most
notable contribution in the area of reinforcement, particularly in
relation to social skills, was made by Skinner (1953), a behavioural
psychologist who pioneered the theory of operant conditioning
(the word 'operant' derives from the fact that the operant
behaviour operates on the environment to produce some effect).
Skinner, working with rats and pigeons, explored the many different effects of reinforcement on behaviour. For example, the rat,
placed in a specially adapted box ('Skinner box') engaged in many
kinds of spontaneous operant behaviour. Eventually the animal,
besides doing other things, pressed a bar. A pellet of food automatically dropped into the feeding cup beneath the bar. Still no
learning took place. In human terms we might say that the animal
did not 'notice' any connection between the food and the bar but
continued its random movements as before. Eventually it pressed
the bar again and another pellet dropped. This time the animal
noticed what had happened and an association was formed
between the act of pressing the bar and reward of food. The rat
now began pressing the bar as fast as it could eat one pellet and get
back to the bar to release another. Thus the presentation of the
food was a positive reinforcement of the bar-pressing behaviour.

Positive reinforcement, therefore, occurs when the presence of a
stimulus strengthens a response. In human terms, the behaviour of
joke telling is a good example. Should we tell a joke at work and our
colleagues laugh, then we might tell the joke again in the company
of different people. Thus the behaviour of joke telling has been
increased. If, however, the audience remain silent we would be
unlikely to tell the joke again. The good consequence (e.g. laughter
at our joke) is called a positive reinforcer or strengthener. Alter-

natively, behaviour can also be encouraged by negatively reinforcing certain responses. Negative reinforcement occurs when the
withdrawal of a stimulus strengthens the tendency to behave in a
certain way. In the previous experiment with the rat, bar pressing
could have been increased by administering a mild electric shock
which could only have been terminated by actually pressing the
bar. Gradually the rat would have performed this piece of
behaviour with increasing frequency in order to have alleviated the
discomfort caused by the electric shock. Again in human terms an
example of such reinforcement can typically be seen in certain
psychiatric patients who have been institutionalised for many
years. If attention is given only when the patient talks incoherently,
neglects hygiene, speaks of hallucinations, or generally acts anti-
socially, the attention, even if negative, reinforces the responses.

Punishment and extinction are two other terms frequently associated with reinforcement. Punishment, unlike negative reinforcement, decreases the frequency of the behaviour under focus.
Extinction, alternatively, occurs when the positive or negative reinforcement used to alter behaviour during operant conditioning is
removed, resulting in the frequency of conditional responses
gradually being reduced to the level that existed prior to the conditioning. The rat, for example, if no longer rewarded with food
would cease pressing the bar (see Figure 9.3). Because both
negative reinforcement and punishment involve aversive stimuli,
their application to social skills is rather restricted. Skinner's
theory, in addition, contends that negative reinforcement merely
produces escape and/or avoidance behaviour.

Variables Affecting Reinforcement

When using reinforcement during social interaction there are many
variables to be taken into consideration.

Type of Reinforcement.   With animals it is relatively easy to provide suitable reinforcement. Food and water constitute an obvious
kind of reward and because of their biological value, are
commonly referred to as primary reinforcers. Additional primary
reinforcers include air, warmth, and sex. Although extremely
strong reinforcers they are not generally used to alter or maintain
behaviour, although they have been used in extreme circumstances
(e.g. in interrogation where a subject is not allowed to eat or sleep
until they agree to a particular demand). Human beings, in every-

Figure 9.3: Effects of Various Stimuli on Behaviour

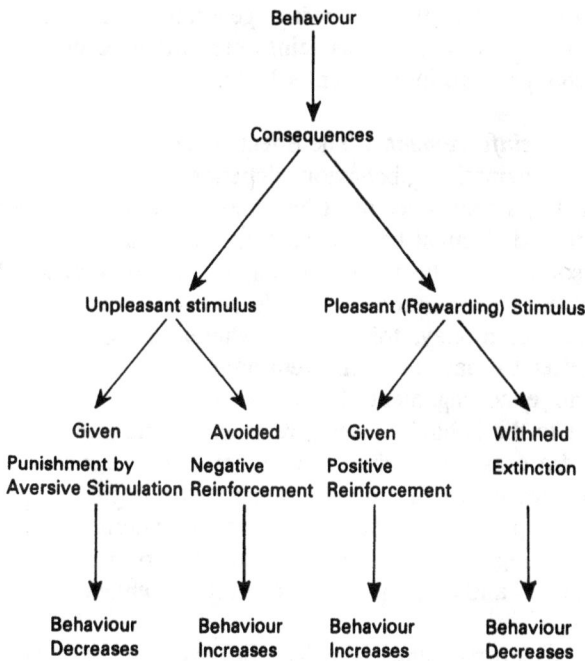

day terms, seldom react in order to receive food, water etc. Instead they usually seem to react to less tangible rewards such as praise or acceptance. These rewards are called secondary reinforcers, and it has been assumed that they have gained their value because of their association with more fundamental concerns such as food.

Timing and Schedules of Reinforcement. The timing of reinforcement has been studied in great detail. A common assumption in training animals or children has been that it is most effective to reward directly after the desirable behaviour occurs. Immediate feedback, therefore, produces the most rapid learning. In addition to timing, the frequency of schedule of reinforcement is also important. Delivery of reinforcement after every occurrence of a response is called continuous reinforcement. Alternatively, occasional delivery of reinforcement is called partial or '*intermittent*' *reinforcement.* Ferster and Skinner (1957) have chronicled the effects of various reinforcement schedules. They discovered that continuous reinforcement will produce a weak habit very quickly, while intermittent reinforcement will produce a strong habit relatively slowly. Hence the following generalisations: to get a behaviour going use continuous reinforcement; to keep it going gradually change to an intermittent schedule.

Appropriate Reinforcement. The effectiveness of a reinforcer in changing and maintaining behaviour depends greatly upon several factors. Firstly, a reinforcer must be of some value to the person being reinforced. It must be remembered that what is reinforcing to one person may not be so for another. Work and domestic skills appear to be more effectively reinforced with more tangible rewards such as money, tokens etc., whereas social behaviours respond better to 'natural' social reinforcers such as recognition, support and encouragement. Secondly, a reinforcer should be appropriate to the behaviour being reinforced. The individual, for example, who uses superlatives such as 'brilliant', 'excellent', etc. to reinforce responses that do not warrant the degree of praise, may appear superficial, sarcastic and even insincere. Conversely insufficient strength in reinforcement may undermine the person being reinforced and consequently affect future behaviour.

Variety of Reinforcement. Finally, the over-use of a specific reinforcer may ultimately lead to loss of its reinforcing properties. Continued use of the same phrase (such as 'well done') following every bit of desirable behaviour becomes monotonous and loses some of its effectiveness. Praise should be varied, using phrases such as 'good', 'great', 'that's terrific', 'you've done very well this time', and sometimes a smile or a nod will do just as well. When using a variety of reinforcers, however, one should bear in mind that alternative reinforcers should be appropriate as discussed in the previous section.

Social Reinforcement

Having taken a cursory look at the theoretical background of reinforcement, cognisance will now be taken of its role in social situations. Acknowledging that a reinforcer can be considered as anything that is positively valued by an individual, one can appreciate that social reinforcers can be many and varied. Only the main elements of social reinforcement, therefore, will be discussed in this section.

Social reinforcers can be described as those behaviours displayed during the normal course of interaction which increase the frequency or improve the quality of a social behaviour it follows. Such reinforcing behaviour may be either verbal or nonverbal in nature.

Verbal Reinforcement. Effective verbal reinforcement can range in complexity from simple monosyllabic expressions such as 'good' or 'fine' to the more complex reflective techniques as discussed earlier in this chapter. One of the simplest ways to reinforce another's behaviour is by merely verbally acknowledging or confirming that listening and agreement have taken place. These responses include a variety of utterances, words and phrases such as 'yes', 'OK', 'sure', 'mm-hmmm', 'that's right' etc. The effects of such social reinforcers on human behaviour have been widely studied. Greenspoon (1955) asked subjects to utter words at random for 50 minutes. Some subjects were reinforced by an 'mm-hmm' or a 'good' for every single noun they generated while others were reinforced only for plural nouns. For both groups, the verbal reinforcement significantly increased the generation rate for the type of word that was rewarded. Centres (1963) studied the control of everyday conversation through the use of simple social reinforcers. While supposedly waiting for an experiment, subjects sat in the waiting room of a psychology department. A confederate of the experimenter (who acted like a subject) joined the real subjects and initiated conversation. Through the use of simple social reinforcers such as utterances and words the confederate was able to influence the total verbalisation of subjects, the number of statements they made conveying information and the number of statements of opinion.

In addition to acknowledging and agreeing with another, stronger verbal reinforcement entails actually encouraging certain behaviours through praise and support. Responses include superlatives and phrases such as 'very good', 'great idea', 'you are doing very well', 'keep at it' etc. This type of social reinforcer indicates that the person providing them not only agrees with, and wants to help, the speaker but also wishes for the other to continue to respond in a particular way. Empirical studies have shown that such social reinforcers can actually affect underlying attitudes and beliefs. Insko (1965), for example, interviewed students by telephone about their feelings toward a proposed festival. Half of the students were reinforced with encouraging statements whenever they expressed feelings of support for the festival. The other half were similarly reinforced for statements opposing the festival. Following a general opinion survey the answers of those who previously had been verbally reinforced for pro-festival statements showed more favourable attitudes toward the festival than did the answers of those who had not received the reinforcements.

Praise and support, therefore, have been shown to be potent social reinforcers, not only in encouraging the speaker to continue talking but also to alter the speaker's responses.

A third, and perhaps even more powerful, form of verbal reinforcement is that of developing and exploring the speaker's responses. The previous two categories, although useful, can be 'performed' at quite a superficial level, whereas the development and exploration of responses through such techniques as questioning (see Chapter 8) and reflection (as discussed earlier in this chapter) can help convey sincerity and genuine interest on the part of the listener. By questioning and reflecting, the listener indicates that he has been attending closely and that the information contained is considered worthy of one's time and effort in order to explore it further.

Nonverbal Reinforcement.   Social reinforcement takes forms other than verbal reinforcement. As discussed in Chapter 7, nonverbal social skills are a potent form of communication and can (because of the difficulty in falsifying them) be a more accurate indication of a person's innermost feelings. For example in situations where the verbal behaviour contradicts the nonverbal message, Shapiro (1968) showed that listeners generally take more credence of the nonverbal behaviour. The use, therefore, of nonverbal reinforcers in social situations is of great importance. Such nonverbal reinforcers include smiling, nodding, increased eye-contact, touch and appropriate posture and proximity.

Functions of Social Reinforcement

Social reinforcers can have both an extrinsic and an intrinsic value to the person providing them. Extrinsically they may help achieve a particular response in another such as increasing appropriate behaviour. Intrinsically they may be associated with popularity, as people who provide appropriate reinforcers are often seen to be warm, friendly and understanding in nature. The most salient functions served by reinforcement as outlined by Hargie et al (1981) include:

(1) To promote interaction and maintain relationships
(2) To increase the involvement of the other person
(3) To encourage the other person to continue to talk about a specific topic
(4) To increase appropriate and decrease inappropriate behaviour
(5) To demonstrate a genuine interest in the ideas, thoughts or feelings expressed by the other
(6) To make interaction enjoyable and rewarding
(7) To create an impression of warmth and understanding.

The inability to reinforce effectively, as seen in many psychiatric patients, can have a detrimental effect on social interaction. Trower et al (1978), for example, identified that certain groups of patients use very little reinforcement during conversation. This may be construed by others as disinterest, distancing and even unfriendliness. Such perceptions can result in the diminution of conversation and ultimately the termination of rapport.

Overview

Four responding skills have been discussed in this chapter, namely: listening, empathising, reflecting and reinforcing. Although for purposes of clarity each has been discussed separately, it should be realised that each skill is closely allied to a number of other social skills. In empathising, for example, one must *listen* attentively to what is said, *reflect* accurately the person's feelings, and *reinforce* appropriately so as to encourage the individual to continue interacting. No one responding skill, therefore, can be seen or practised in isolation from the rest.

Many such responding skills are affected by psychiatric illness. The degree to which they are affected varies markedly from one illness to the next, ranging from total unresponsiveness in the chronic schizophrenic to the psychopathic person who responds quite effectively — albeit for manipulative purposes. Since many of the problems in the re-socialisation of patients centres around their inability to respond appropriately during interaction, enhancing these skills, through techniques such as SST, *must* be an integral part of the rehabilitatory process.

10 SST EXERCISES

In this chapter we describe a number of SST exercises that can be employed with psychiatric patients. However, these should be treated as ideas upon which to build more specific exercises geared specifically to meet the needs of particular patient groups. It is certainly not our intention to present a cook-book approach to SST, since the form and the content of this training method have to be tailored to the requirements of different patients. As such, we would recommend that the nurse should gradually develop methods and exercises found to be successful with particular patient populations. These methods and exercises may come from a number of sources. Indeed, one social skills text recommends: 'Another principle we have borrowed, and which will become apparent as the book proceeds, is that of *plagiarism*. Workers on the lookout for materials to use in the way proposed here will soon find that the environment is full of them. We advocate the adoption of a "jackdaw" attitude towards anything at all that may be of value for particular programmes' (Priestley et al, 1978). In other words, those involved in SST should be prepared to adapt available materials to suit their own requirements. It is in this spirit that we present a number of suggested exercises for each of the social skills described in this book, based upon our own experiences of conducting SST programmes.

Nonverbal Communication

This skill lends itself to a wide variety of different types of exercise during SST. To sensitise patients to the entire area of nonverbal communication, a useful starting point is to show them a video recording of an interaction, with the sound turned down, and ask them to comment upon the nature of the interaction taking place and the behaviour of those involved. This serves as a useful warm-up exercise with which to introduce this field of study.

For particular aspects of nonverbal communication, different exercises can be employed. To analyse facial expressions photographs are very useful and these can be easily produced by the nurse, or existing photographs in books can be used (e.g. Spence, 1980). Similarly, photographs can also be used to analyse different postures, although matchstick-men illustrations can also be employed. The effects of orientation and proximity can be emphasised by asking patients to arrange a room for a specific purpose (e.g. a selection interview) and having patients indicate where they would stand or sit. In relation to touch, patients can be asked to produce lists of when it would be appropriate to touch, or be touched by, others, and where they would be touched. To facilitate this, a list can be drawn up as follows:

PERSON	PART OF BODY TOUCHED
Mother	
Father	
Close male friend	
Close female friend	
Someone just introduced	
Complete stranger	
Doctor	

Paralanguage can best be focused upon by using an audio-recorder. One technique here is to record a neutral message in several ways emphasising different types of emotion through the use of paralanguage (anger, excitement, sadness etc.). Patients can then be asked to listen to each of these and identify the type of emotion being portrayed. The nurse can also use short excerpts from TV programmes or video films (copyright permitting) to illustrate elements of nonverbal communication. Failing this, it is relatively simple to set up and video-record a number of short scenarios depicting nonverbal behaviours. All that is needed is a video-recorder, a TV camera, a few volunteer actors, and a little imagination!

At a later stage patients should be actively involved in encoding nonverbal signals. For example, the patient can be given a piece of paper on which is described an emotion which they then have to convey to the group through facial expression and/or posture. Patients should also, where appropriate, be involved in role plays which are video recorded. These can then be replayed without sound to underline the patient's nonverbal behaviour, or without vision to emphasise paralanguage. However, the importance of synchronisation of nonverbal behaviour and vocals should be high-lighted where necessary, and the tape played back with both sound and vision present.

Self-disclosure

Who I Am

This exercise is designed as a warm-up for the analysis and practice of the skill of self-disclosure. The purpose here is to encourage patients to think about themselves more deeply. The first step is to ask patients to complete a list of 20 descriptors which they would use to describe themselves. The patient should be given complete freedom to produce this list, although basic examples might be given (e.g. name, married or single). Thus, they fill in a sheet headed Who I Am and numbered (1) to (20) as a list on the left-hand side, for the patient to put their descriptors against. These 20 descriptors can then be categorised into six main areas:

(1) Physical factors: These provide some indication of how the patient 'sees himself'. Examples include: tall, thin, blonde, male, white, bald.
(2) Identifying 'tags': These would include name, address and nationality.
(3) Habits and practices: These are recurring patterns of behaviour displayed by the individual including: smoker, jogger, heavy drinker, car-driver.
(4) Personality and temperament: This relates to the type of person that the patient sees themselves as being. Descriptors used here would include quiet, conscientious, friendly, aggressive, open, lively.
(5) Social roles. These descriptors focus upon the roles patients play in society, such as: husband, wife, father, plumber, teacher.
(6) Beliefs, attitudes and values. These relate to the ideals each individual holds, and would include descriptors such as: socialist, anti-apartheid, Christian, Jew.

These aspects of identity can then be discussed with the patient, and evaluated in four ways:

(1) Saliency: How important is each aspect for the patient? Which descriptors were used initially? Which types of descriptor were used most frequently? These factors provide further insight into how the patient views himself.
(2) Stability: How stable are each of the aspects of identity? How many descriptors has the patient control over? Which ones might they want to change?
(3) Valence: This is the degree to which each aspect of identity is viewed as positive or negative by the patient. Which descriptors are positive and which are negative? Overall, are there more positive than negative descriptors?
(4) Utility: How useful are each of the aspects of identity in terms of the goals of the patient? Which descriptors facilitate the achievement of these goals, and which make their achievement more difficult?

Depth of Self-disclosure

In order to encourage the patient to consider this element, produce a list of disclosures (such as below) and have patients sort these out in order of high, medium or low levels of depth, if told to a complete stranger.

DISCLOSURE	DEPTH LEVEL (HIGH, MEDIUM OR LOW)
I am tired	
My name is John	
I am an alcoholic	
I am 24 years old	
I am divorced	
I killed a man when I was 18	
I am a plumber	
I like being on my own most of the time	
Sometimes I feel like ending it all	
I was born in Belfast	
I am undergoing psychiatric treatment	
I think you are sexy	
I have athlete's foot	

> I think I no longer love my
>   wife
> I detest socialists
> I like pop music
> I am a vegetarian
> My mother died last week
> I have been unemployed for
>   2 years
> I am homeless
> I am really depressed

Targets for Self-disclosure

To encourage patients to consider what type of disclosure to make to different people, produce a list of people (as below) and get patients to sort out the types of disclosure they would make to each (the disclosure statements listed on the 'Depth of Self-disclosure' exercise can be used here as an alternative to the Disclosure Types).

TARGET
Spouse
Work-mate
Close friend
Mother
Complete stranger (same sex)
Complete stranger (opposite sex)
Father
Acquaintance
Son
Daughter
Nurse

DISCLOSURE TYPES
Minor health problems (sore throat, sprained ankle)
Embarrassing personal history (jail sentence, psychiatric problems etc.)
Descriptive personal details (name, age etc.)
Shallow feelings (like, enjoy etc.)
Deep feelings (love, hate etc.)
Embarrassing health problems (V.D., haemorrhoids etc.)
Major health problems (cancer, Parkinson's disease etc.)

Personal problems (unemployed, separated etc.)
Personal aspirations (to get married, get promotion)

The final stage should involve role-plays in which patients are required to self-disclose. These can be recorded and then replayed with appropriate feedback on performance.

Greetings and Partings

As a warm up, patients should be asked to write down as many words or phrases as they can which are used during greetings and partings. These should then be called out, and written down on a blackboard by the nurse, to underline the emphasis given to this element in everyday social interaction. A similar exercise can be completed in terms of the nonverbal behaviours associated with greetings and partings. Patients should also be asked to think of as many different functions as they can for going through the rituals of greeting and parting. As before, these can then be listed on the blackboard to stimulate further interest in this area of study.

Again, it is useful to show patients video recordings of greetings and partings in different settings, and as mentioned earlier these can either be short snippets taken from TV programmes and video films, or can be self-produced. The exemplars used should, of course, link directly to areas that patients find difficult, be it dating, meeting strangers or whatever. These video exemplars serve as useful models, and also help to stimulate detailed discussion and analysis. Finally, role-plays can be enacted of different types of greetings and partings, with accompanying video recording and feedback. The skill of self-disclosure then can be integrated within the analysis of greetings.

Asking Questions

This topic can be introduced by asking patients to give a definition of 'a question'. This focuses attention upon the area of information gathering, and this attention can be further stimulated by having patients identify as many functions or purposes for questions as they can. These functions should be listed on the blackboard to highlight the variety of reasons why questions are asked. At this stage, patients should be motivated to learn more about the different types of questions that can be asked, and their likely effects.

The use of audio or video-taped models is vital to illustrate the skill of questioning in action. Models should initially be used to help patients identify each type of question separately. This can then be followed by taped sequences incorporating various types of questions, during which patients attempt to identify each question and evaluate its effectiveness.

In group SST, a useful exercise is to divide the group into sub-groups, and have each sub-group produce a transcript of an interaction in which a number of questions are employed. Each sub-group then takes turns to 'enact' the transcript for the other sub-groups, but the interaction stops after each question and the other sub-groups try to identify the question and evaluate its appropriateness. This exercise involves patients actively generating as well as evaluating questions.

Finally, role-plays should be conducted and recorded with each patient given an opportunity to ask questions in specific simulated situations. This can then be followed by detailed feedback and analysis of the questioning skills of each patient.

Explaining

As with the skill of questioning, patients can be asked to offer definitions of the term 'explanation', and identify the main functions of this skill in social interaction. Once a definition has been agreed upon and the function outlined, a useful exercise is to divide the group into sub-groups and give each sub-group a card bearing the name of a concept which they have to explain to the other groups. The sub-groups should be given several minutes to work out an appropriate explanation for their concept (with the proviso that they do not mention the concept itself!) A spokesperson from each sub-group then presents the explanation to the other groups, who try to ascertain what the concept is. This exercise will underline for patients the importance of effective explanation, and will also serve as an introduction to some of the behaviours associated with the skill of explaining. The concepts employed in this exercise will depend upon the ability level of the patients but may include terms such as: aggression; authority; backward; hopeful; kindness; wonderful.

Specific situations where patients will need to give explanations should be explored (e.g. at selection interviews), and where possible audio or video-taped models should be shown. As before, nurses should endeavour to produce model tapes, geared specifically to meet the needs of their own target group and the context in which these groups operate. This should then be followed by practicals in which patients are given an opportunity to present explanations in specific role-play settings, and provided with appropriate feedback on their performance.

Assertiveness

The methods used during the analysis of assertiveness will depend upon the patients and the situations in which they find it difficult to be assertive. However, some general procedures can be applied. The first of these is to identify as many situations as possible that cause assertion problems for patients. Each of these should then be studied separately, with patients being encouraged to identify what the rights of the people involved in each situation are. This is important, since patients may hold mistaken beliefs about their rights, and therefore these need to be fully discussed before moving on to examine assertive behaviour. Unless inappropriate cognitions are overcome, skills training in assertiveness is likely to be unsuccessful.

The next step is to present to patients the continuum of:
Non-assertion ——————— Assertion ——————— Aggression.
Each of these styles of responding should be explained in terms of their behavioural components, and patients should be given examples of how each style can be used as a response to the same situation, and of their probable effects. Thus, patients would be presented with three alternative responses to a given situation, as below.

When queueing to get into the cinema someone walks right in front of you rather than going to the end of the queue. Consider the following alternative responses:
(1) You feel aggrieved but say nothing, in the hope that someone else will confront the queue jumper
(2) You grab the person by the arm and say 'Hey you, get to the back of the queue!'

(3) You say to the person 'Excuse me, but do you realise there is a queue here and the end of the line is further back'.

Here (1) is non-assertive, (2) is aggressive and (3) is assertive. Numerous further examples of these three styles can be found in Alberti and Emmons (1975, 1982) and Lange and Jakubowski (1976), and these texts also contain assertiveness tests as well as a great deal of useful material for trainers.

Patients should then be given hypothetical situations and asked to generate non-assertive, aggressive and assertive responses. This can best be achieved by again using the sub-group technique, wherein two or three individuals come together to discuss issues and then report back to the overall group. This encourages maximum participation. Each sub-group should then have an opportunity to display their three alternative responses (using a blackboard, flip-chart etc.) to the full group and discuss the relative merits and demerits of each response.

Video-taped exemplars of assertive, non-assertive and aggressive responses should be shown. These can be made fairly easily, and it is more effective if they are tailor-made to meet the situations that patients find difficult. Following this modelling stage, patients should engage in role-plays of situations in which assertiveness is necessary. The different forms of assertiveness outlined in Chapter 8 should be practised by patients, beginning with role-plays that are not too difficult or threatening, and gradually escalating the degree of difficulty as the confidence of the patient increases.

Interacting in Groups

In a sense, the entire SST programme contributes towards the ability of the patient to interact in groups, since either such training takes place in a group, or at least the patient will have to interact with the nurse and other professionals where training is individualised. However, while involvement in such groups will be valuable for patients, some more direct attempt should also be made to improve the ability of patients to interact in a group situation. At the same time, since this will be a very difficult area for many patients, great care and sensitivity needs to be exercised to ensure that no patient suffers unduly during group exercises.

The analysis of group interaction can begin by having patients discuss the main functions of groups as outlined in Chapter 8. This should be followed by an evaluation of the effects (positive and negative) which groups have upon individuals, and of why some individuals are more successful than others in group interactions. This can be exemplified by showing video-tapes of group discussions and having patients discuss the performance of each group member.

Patients should then be involved in actively participating in a group exercise, which can be video-taped and then played back for detailed feedback and evaluation. This group exercise can take various forms. One approach is to give patients a topic or topics to discuss, and record the discussion. Another approach is to give patients a task to complete (e.g. cut up three large photographs into smaller pieces and put all of the pieces into a large envelope; present the envelope to the group, who are told simply that the pieces should be reassembled but are not informed that the pieces represent three separate photographs) and record the group at work. A third approach is to give each group member a task to complete individually and then complete the same task as a group. This latter approach can be used to analyse the ability of patients to influence a group, or the extent to which they can be led by others. For example, patients can be presented with a list of 15 items and asked to rank order these individually. Then a number of patients attempt to come to an agreement as a group about the rank ordering of these items.

In the example presented below, the 15 items are human needs. In Step One patients only complete the column marked 'O.R.' (Own Ranking) individually. The next stage of the exercise is to move to Step Two and have a group of patients come together and complete the column marked 'G.R.' (Group Ranking) by coming to a group agreement about each item. The grid system is used to allow group members to compare one another's scores easily. This part of the exercise should be video-recorded. Finally, patients complete Step Three by filling in the column marked 'O.R.2' (Own Ranking, Second Occasion) individually. Once all of these rankings have been obtained, scores can be tabulated as below.

Step One Page

Have patients insert the group ranking scores in the 'G.R.' column. Then for each item subtract the lower score from the higher score

NEEDS EXERCISE I

STEP ONE   INSTRUCTIONS   NAME_____

Below are listed 15 types of human needs. Your task is to evaluate each, in terms of their importance for the average individual in our society. Place the number 1 by the most important need, the number 2 by the second most important need, and so on through to number 15, the least important need. Think carefully about your reasons for these rankings, since you will have to present these reasons in the next step of this exercise when you will have to come to a group consensus about the rankings. At this stage, however, you should complete the column marked 'O.R.' individually.

	O.R.	G.R.	Change
Pain avoidance			
Friends			
Food			
Self-respect			
Air			
Esteem of others			
Sex			
Children			
Achievement			
Water			
Exercise			
Security			
A mate			
Stability			
Rest			

TOTAL_____

NEEDS EXERCISE II

STEP TWO   INSTRUCTIONS   NAME_____

Now that each individual in your group has rank-ordered the 15 individual items your next step is to reach a group consensus about the ordering. This means that the prediction for each of the 15 individual items *must* be agreed upon by each member before it becomes part of the group decision. Consensus is difficult to reach, therefore not every ranking will meet with everyone's complete approval. Try, as a group, to make each ranking one with which *all* group members can at least partially agree.

Try to: (1) Avoid arguing solely for your own individual judgements. Approach the task on the basis of logic.

(2) Avoid changing your mind just to reach agreement and avoid conflict. Support only those solutions with which you can at least agree in part.

(3) View differences of opinion as helpful rather than as hindrances.

(4) View your initial agreement as suspect.

	1	2	3	4	5	6	7	8	G.R.
Pain avoidance									
Friends									
Food									
Self-respect									
Air									
Esteem of others									
Sex									
Children									
Achievement									
Water									
Exercise									
Security									
A mate									
Stability									
Rest									

NEEDS EXERCISE III

STEP THREE INSTRUCTIONS NAME_____

Complete this part of the exercise individually. We are interested in your final
judgement of the 15 types of needs. Again, your task is to evaluate in terms of their
importance for the average individual in our society. Place the number 1 by the most
important need, the number 2 by the second most important need and so on through to
number 15 the least important need. At this stage, complete the column marked O.R.2.

	O.R.2	O.R.1	O.R. Change
Pain avoidance			
Friends			
Food			
Self-respect			
Air			
Esteem of others			
Sex			
Children			
Achievement			
Water			
Exercise			
Security			
A mate			
Stability			
Rest			

TOTAL_____

and insert the difference in the 'Change' column. Ignore sign differences (i.e. do not have minus scores). For example:

	O.R.	G.R.	Change
Pain avoidance	10	4	6
Friends	5	14	9

Then add up all the individual change scores to get a total change score. The higher this change score total, the more likely it is that the individual has been influenced by the group.

Step Three Page

Insert the O.R.1 (Own Ranking, First Occasion) scores and, again, for each item subtract the lower from the higher score and insert the difference in the O.R. change column. As before, add up all of the change scores to get a total O.R. change score. The higher this score the more the individual has really been influenced by the views of group members. However, if this score is low, but the O.R./G.R. change total is high, this would suggest that the patient has acquiesed in the group without actually being convinced about the decisions being taken.

The scores obtained from this type of exercise provide valuable information to complement the analysis of the video-recording of the group interaction. As emphasised earlier, however, the nurse must be very sensitive about how such information is utilised.

Listening

As a way of introduction, patients should be asked to define what is meant by the term, focusing particularly on 'active' as opposed to 'passive' listening. As outlined in Chapter 9, aspects including the verbal and nonverbal variety of responses in listening should then be identified. These can be listed on a blackboard or flipchart and discussed, highlighting the variety of responses that exist.

As one must 'listen' to the nonverbal as well as the verbal message, exercises discussed in the nonverbal section may be employed here. Such exercises can include the use of video-taped conversations, recorded either from the TV network or compiled by oneself. Firstly, by turning down the sound, patients should 'listen' to the nonverbal messages being conveyed. Similarly by turning up the sound and blackening out the picture, patients can be asked to identify, by focusing on paralanguage, the meanings being portrayed. Following patient feedback and discussion on the above exercises, a video-taped model proficient in the art of listening may demonstrate the skill in action. Different listening skill components may initially be presented separately (e.g. eye contact, posture, types of verbal response) and analysed. This can then be followed by taped sequences depicting a combination of listening skills used during conversation. These tapes may be used to stimulate discussion and consolidate what has already been covered.

Based on the knowledge of what constitutes effective listening, patients should be divided up into groups of three. Each is ascribed a specific role namely speaker, listener and observer. The speaker talks about something which is of common interest (e.g. holidays) while the listener seeks to illustrate an appropriate range of listening behaviours. The observer watches the listener's efforts closely. After a specified time the observer comments on the listener's skills. The speaker may also contribute their feelings about the listener's feedback during conversation. Each member of the group then changes roles and the sequence is repeated until all have played each of the three roles. This exercise is particularly useful initially, allowing patients to practise listening skills in small groups before graduating to larger audiences or CCTV. It also affords other members of the group the opportunity to analyse critically what is going on. In certain situations, however, the psychiatric nurse may work solely with the patient, playing the part of the speaker. This may occur where a patient objects to working with other patients or where individual patient's problems require specific attention and feedback. Following the role-play exercises, groups can come together and contribute to an overall feedback session.

In the final exercise, patients should participate in role play situations. These can be recorded and played back, focusing on specific problems if necessary. It is important that the patient is allowed to practise skills and is appropriately supported and reinforced by nursing staff.

Reflection

Following a short video recording of an interaction, patients should be asked to comment on the messages being conveyed, namely facts and feelings. Having differentiated between the two, the steps in and functions of reflection (as discussed in the previous chapter) should then be identified and listed on a blackboard or flip-chart to aid clarity.

As one of the initial steps in reflection of feeling is the identification of emotions expressed, it is imperative that the patient is able to perceive accurately the speaker's feelings. A useful exercise to determine this, as detailed by Spence (1980), is through the use of photographs depicting different expressions and postures. The patient's ability to label accurately the emotions contained in each expression and posture will help indicate their sensitivity and perceptiveness of another's feelings. Similarly, audiotapes and videotapes can be used to present the patient with a variety of voice quality and gesture cues (see exercise below). The patient is given a list of emotions and asked to label each emotion played accordingly. An extension of this exercise may entail patients role-playing certain emotions to others, who in turn must determine what they are.

In addition to perceiving accurately the other's feelings, effective reflection requires the patient to translate the speaker's message into his own words ensuring the same level of intensity and including certain paraphrased elements of the speaker's past statement. This may be illustrated through the use of a video-taped model, pausing if necessary to focus on and emphasise certain points.

Written statements can also be given to patients who are asked to devise an appropriate reflection for each statement. Similarly, a video-taped statement can be presented and patients asked to write down their reflections. These can then be discussed, taking cognisance of the requisites mentioned above. Finally, sub-groups can be formed with the purpose of one reflecting the other's statements. These may be recorded and replayed with appropriate feedback on performance. Again, as mentioned earlier, it is imperative that appropriate responses are reinforced by the nurse therapist.

EXERCISE I

Perception of Emotional Expression from Voice Quality Cues

NAME ....

INSTRUCTIONS

The following method is suggested for assessing the ability to perceive the meaning of emotional voice quality cues.

> You are going to hear a tape of a person talking. The words don't mean anything but each sounds as if the person is feeling a particular emotion or feeling. I will give you a choice of five feelings to choose from. Now listen carefully to the first voice. (The nurse then plays the first emotion)
> 'Does that person sound happy, bored, sad, angry, or frightened?'
> The tape may be played once and the choice repeated once if no response is made to each question. The instructions are repeated in the same way for all the subsequent voices. The scores can then be totalled.

	ORDER OF PRESENTATION AND CORRECT RESPONSE	SCORE
VOICE	A. ANGRY B. SAD C. BORED D. HAPPY E. FRIGHTENED	
	TOTAL SCORE	

Correct response — 1
Incorrect or no response after one repetition — 0

Empathy

Many of the aforementioned skills are used in the empathetic process. Social skills including active listening, reflecting content and feeling, appropriate posture, eye contact, touch, paralanguage etc., are necessary prerequisites for effective empathising. Training a patient to empathise more effectively, therefore, involves focusing on one skill at a time, devising programmes that will allow a degree of competency to be achieved in each. Information relating to individual empathetic components (e.g. listening, reflecting) were reviewed earlier in this chapter. In addition the following exercises may prove useful in enhancing one's empathising potential.

The topic can be introduced by presenting and discussing the meaning and characteristics of empathy. Later this may be broadened to differentiate between empathy and sympathy. Awareness of the subject may be further heightened by guiding the patient to read relevant background material.

Once a basic understanding of the concept has been acquired the patient should be shown a video-taped model demonstrating various empathetic responses. Situations demonstrated by the model should, where possible, depict circumstances pertinent to the patient's own lifestyle. To assist critical analysis of the model's performance an empathetic rating scale may be used. Nelson-Jones (1982), for example, suggested the following:

5 = Very good empathetic response
4 = Good empathetic response
3 = Moderate empathetic response
2 = Slight empathy in the response
1 = Response not at all empathetic

Once the patient has rated the model's performance, discussion should follow as to why each rating was given.

In group SST patients can then be sub-divided into pairs. In extenuating circumstances the patient may work solely with the nurse therapist. Individual empathetic skills can be enacted with each person taking turns to role play both the speaker and empathising listener. Role play exercises to enhance nonverbal empathetic behaviour, for example, may include those for seating position, body position and seating and body position together.

Seating Position

(1) Distance. You sit in a chair and listen to your partner talking: (a) with your heads 18 inches apart; (b) with your heads 6-8 feet apart. Then start moving in until your partner says it feels a comfortable distance. You and your partner then reverse roles, followed by discussion.
(2) Height. Your partner talks and you listen while you: (a) sit in a noticeably higher chair; (b) sit in a noticeably lower chair; and (c) sit in a chair of the same height. You and your partner reverse roles, then discuss.
(3) Angle. Your partner talks and you listen while: (a) sitting squarely opposite so that your right shoulder is directly across

from your partner's left shoulder; (b) sitting at 90 degrees so that the front of your chair faces the right side of your partner's chair. Then move your chair until your partner indicates this to be a comfortable angle. You and your partner reverse roles, then discuss.

Body Position

(1) Posture. Both seated, your partner talks and you listen while you: (a) have your arms and legs tightly crossed; (b) sprawl loosely in your chair; and (c) try to adopt a relaxed and attentive posture. You and your partner reverse roles, then discuss.

(2) Trunk Lean. Both seated, your partner talks and you listen while you: (a) lean right back; (b) lean far forward; and (c) lean slightly forward. You and your partner reverse roles, then discuss.

(3) Eye Contact. Both seated, your partner talks and you listen while you: (a) avoid your partner's gaze altogether; (b) stare at your partner; and (c) maintain good eye contact, yet look away every now and then. You and your partner reverse roles, then discuss.

Seating and Body Position

(1) Your partner talks for a few minutes while you listen in a correct seating position and combining a relaxed posture, slight forward trunk lean and good eye contact. You and your partner reverse roles, then discuss.

The format of the above exercise can be used to enhance other empathetic skills such as paralanguage. The above may be recorded and played back to other group members. This can facilitate detailed analysis of each skill enacted. Finally appropriate responses by the patient should be suitably reinforced by the nurse therapist.

Reinforcement

In social reinforcement, like empathy, many different social skills are employed. Social reinforcement may include nonverbal behaviours such as nodding, smiling, increased eye contact, posture, touch and verbal responses ranging from monosyllabic replies to questioning and reflecting techniques.

Training exercises to enhance an individual's reinforcing technique necessitate looking at each individual reinforcing behaviour in turn. Comprehensive assessment allows training to be geared towards those areas in which the patient experiences problems. As with empathy, information concerning individual reinforcing skills (e.g. questioning, nonverbal behaviours) can be reviewed as in earlier chapters. In addition the following format may be useful in enhancing one's reinforcing potential.

Sub-groups of three can be used to assess and improve reinforcement technique through a practice-observation-feedback cycle. One member role-plays the speaker, one the listener who demonstrates reinforcing behaviour and the third the observer who gives feedback on the listener's reinforcing abilities. The patient demonstrating reinforcing behaviour should be observed with emphasis being placed on the degree to which he is rewarding or reinforcing the person he is trying to help. For this purpose the observer should look, as suggested by Priestley and McGuire (1983), for the following types of behaviour:

(1) Paying attention. The most fundamental kind of reward you can give a person is just showing them that you are interested in what they have to say.
(2) Reflecting feeling. Conveying to someone that you understand and endorse their feelings is an ingredient of reinforcement.
(3) Use of reinforcers. Observers should record the frequency and appropriateness of nods, smiles, use of the word 'yes' and other verbal and nonverbal components of social reinforcement.
(4) Emphasis on positive statements. By extracting and focusing on the positive elements in what someone has said, mentioning their good qualities etc., one can build up positive self-attitudes in those whose views of themselves may initially be somewhat limited or deprecating.

In addition to the observer commenting on the patient's reinforcing technique, the speaker may also explain how they felt about the reinforcement emitted. Following discussion the roles are changed until all parts have been enacted. The above may be video-taped and played back, assisting one to focus on specific aspects of reinforcement.

Overview

Several exercises have been described in this chapter which may help enhance specific social skills in patients. At the expense of repeating ourselves the need to design individualised SST programmes is of paramount importance if success is to be gained. Not only do differences occur from one particular group of patients to another, but they may also exist within groups. Comprehensive assessment is therefore imperative, enabling programmes to be drawn up which will meet, more accurately, the specific needs of the patient.

It is hoped that the examples contained within this text will serve to both orientate and stimulate nurses regarding the types of exercise that can usefully be employed during SST.

11 CONCLUSION

The social skills approach to the remediation of social deficits has gathered increasing momentum during the past decade, and it is important for the psychiatric nurse to be *au fait* with SST techniques and procedures in order to make a contribution to this training method. It is also useful for the nurse to be aware of some of the problems and difficulties involved in implementing SST programmes. To underline both the main facets and the associated difficulties of planning and running such programmes, the following points should be borne in mind:

(1) Careful selection of patients is vital. Some patients will not benefit from SST for a variety of reasons (see Chapter 2), and it is therefore important that patients who have the ability and the motivation to benefit are selected. Otherwise, the programme is likely to be unsuccessful and will be a waste of time for everyone concerned. In particular, patients must have the cognitive capacity to assimilate social skills information.

(2) The full co-operation of patients is crucial. Time spent agreeing the objectives of SST and encouraging the patient to participate fully during training is time well spent. The emphasis should be upon explaining SST as a joint venture in which the patient is an active participant, rather than a passive recipient.

(3) The skills programme should be carefully planned and tailored to meet the identified needs of patients. This means that a detailed assessment of the nature of the patient's social deficits is required (see Chapter 5). Decisions will also have to be made about whether the programme should be individualised or group-based (see Chapter 6). Similarly, decisions will need to be made about how much time to devote to the programme as a whole, and to elements thereof; about whether to use CCTV and/or audio-recordings; and about how to organise practice and feedback sessions.

(4) Be prepared to fight for resources. Since not all staff will either know about, or indeed be in favour of, the SST approach, a marketing task is often required to convince others of its value.

The more resources available for SST, the easier it becomes to implement successful programmes. However, facilities such as time, space and CCTV equipment usually need to be fought for! This can be especially difficult when there is opposition to the introduction of such an 'innovation'. The nurse should be prepared to argue that, in fact, SST is now a tried and tested form of remediation rather than a 'new-fangled craze' which is likely to disappear as quickly as it appeared.

(5) SST usually necessitates a team approach in which the nurse will work closely with other professionals. For this reason, it is imperative that the nurse has a sound understanding of the principles and practice of SST so that they can operate on an equal footing with the psychologist, occupational therapist etc. during training.

(6) The nurse should be socially skilled and sensitive to the social needs of patients during SST. Since modelling is an important component of training, the nurse should be aware that they will be expected to act as a skilled model for patients. If the nurse is lacking in social skills, then the patient is likely to have less confidence in the training approach. Similarly, patients should not be subjected to undue stress or anxiety. To circumvent such problems, practicals and feedback sessions should be carefully structured and closely monitored, so that action can be taken to eliminate possible causes of stress (see Chapter 5).

(7) Particular attention must be devoted to encouraging the generalisation and retention of social skills by patients following training. Programmes that concentrate on these matters tend to produce significant long-term changes in patient behaviour. In particular, the use of a range of personnel and of situations during practicals, the completion of homework assignments, the relevance of SST content to the social difficulties faced by clients, and ensuring that the programme is of sufficient duration to allow for learning, are all useful techniques for promoting transfer. Where possible, follow-up or 'booster' sessions should be organised several months following the SST programme, to stimulate the patient, and consolidate the learning that has taken place.

(8) Always obtain some form of evaluation as to how successful the programme has been. This evaluation can either be formal or informal (see Chapter 6), since either will serve as a necessary feedback mechanism, providing information which

will enable the nurse to make any relevant changes in the nature or content of SST for future patients.

By following these general guidelines, the nurse can help to ensure that SST is as effective as possible in providing benefits for the patient. With proper planning, implementation and follow-up, SST is undoubtedly a very potent tool, which has been shown to be effective in improving the social competence of psychiatric patients. However, as with all training programmes, success requires effort and attention to detail.

SST is therefore a training method with which the psychiatric nurse should be familiar. The potential for this method has been summarised by Christoff and Kelly (1985) who point out that:

Psychiatric patients represent a population for whom social skills training is often useful and appropriate. Building from the clinical studies already conducted, it should be possible for pro-jects to become even more effective and capable of enhancing the interpersonal adjustment of these clients. The future appears promising for clinical interventions, for applied research, and for the improved functioning of patients who receive this training.

We would hope that the information contained in this book will encourage psychiatric nurses to become centrally involved in the provision of SST for as wide a range of patients as possible. We would also point out that while this book provides an overview of SST theory and practice, for a deeper understanding of this approach the nurse should pursue some of the references employed in each chapter. By accumulating as much information as possible the nurse will become a more competent and confident trainer in SST.

REFERENCES

Alberti, R. and Emmons, M. (1975) *Stand Up, Speak Out, Talk Back: The Key to Assertive Behaviour.* Impact, San Luis Obispo, California
— (1982) *Your Perfect Right: A Guide to Assertive Living,* 4th edn. Impact, San Luis Obispo, California
Altschul, A. (1964) 'Group Dynamics and Nursing Care'. *International Journal of Nursing Studies. 1,* 151
Annett, J. (1969) *Feedback and Human Behaviour.* Penguin, Harmondsworth
Argyle, M. (1972) *The Psychology of Interpersonal Behaviour.* 2nd edn. Penguin, Harmondsworth
— and Kendon, A. (1967) 'The Experimental Analysis of Social Performance' in L. Berkowitz (ed) *Advances in Experimental Social Psychology: Volume 3.* Academic Press, New York
—, Furnham, A. and Graham, J. (1981) *Social Situations.* Cambridge University Press, Cambridge
—, Trower, P. and Bryant, B. (1974) 'Explorations in the Treatment of Personality Disorders and Neurosis by Social Skills Training'. *British Journal of Medical Psychology, 47,* 63-72
Arvey, R. and Campion, J. (1984) 'Person Perception in the Employment Interview' in M. Cook (ed) *Issues in Person Perception.* Methuen, London
Athos, A.G. and Gabarro, J.J. (1978) *Interpersonal Behaviour. Communication and Understanding in Relationships.* Prentice-Hall, New Jersey
Averill, J. (1975) 'A Semantic Atlas of Emotional Concepts'. *JSAS Catalogue of Selected Documents in Psychology, 5,* 330
Bandura, A. (1967) 'The Role of Modelling Processes in Personality Development' in T. Foley, R. Lockhart and D. Merrick (eds) *Contemporary Readings in Psychology.* Harper and Row, New York
— (1969) *Principles of Behaviour Modification.* Holt, Rinehart and Winston, New York
— (1971) *Social Learning Theory.* General Learning Press, Morristown, New Jersey
Barton, R. (1976) *Institutional Neurosis,* 3rd edn. Stonebridge Press, John Wright, Bristol
Beckmann-Murray, R. and Wilson-Huelskoetter, M. (1983) *Psychiatric/Mental Health Nursing. Giving Emotional Care.* Prentice-Hall, New Jersey
Becvar, R.J. (1974) *Skills for Effective Communication. A Guide to Building Relationships.* John Wiley & Sons Inc, New York, London
Bernstein, B. (1961) 'Social Structure, Language and Learning' *Educational Research, 3,* 163-176
— (1971) *Class Codes and Control.* Routledge and Kegan Paul, London
Bird, J., Marks, I.M. and Lindley, P. (1979) 'Nurse Therapists in Psychiatry: Developments, Controversies and Implications'. *British Journal of Psychiatry, 135,* 321-329
Birdwhistell, R. (1970) *Kinesics and Context.* University of Pennsylvania Press, Philadelphia
Blondis, M.N. and Jackson, B.E. (1977) *Nonverbal Communication with Patients. Back to the Human Touch.* A Wiley Medical Publication, New York
Brammer, L. (1979) *The Helping Relationship.* Prentice-Hall, New Jersey
Briggs, K. and Wright, B. (1982) 'A Fundamental Skill ... The Aims of and Need

for a Programme of Interpersonal Skills.' *Nursing Mirror, Sep. 1,* 155; 34-6
Bruner, J. and Tagiuri, R. (1954) 'The Perception of People' in C. Lindzey (ed) *Handbook of Social Psychology.* Addison-Wesley, Reading, Mass
Bryant, P.E. (1974) *Perception and Understanding in Young Children.* Methuen, London
Bull, P. (1983) *Body Movement and Interpersonal Communication.* Wiley, Chichester
Butler, R.J. and Rosenthall, G. (1978) *Behaviour and Rehabilitation.* John Wright, Bristol
Centres, R. (1963) 'Laboratory Adaption of the Controversial Procedure for the Conditioning of Verbal Operants.' *Journal of Abnormal and Social Psychology,* 67, 334-379
Christoff, K. and Kelly, J. (1985) 'A Behavioural Approach to Social Skills Training with Psychiatric Patients' in L. L'Abate and M. Milan (eds) *Handbook of Social Skills Training and Research.* Wiley, New York
Cook, M. (1977) 'The Social Skills Model and Interpersonal Attraction' in S. Duck (ed) *Theory and Practice in Interpersonal Attraction.* Academic Press, London
— (1979) *Perceiving Others.* Methuen, London
Coombe, E.I., Jabbusch, B.J., Jones, M.C., Pesznecker, B.L., Ruff, C.M. and Young, K.J. (1981) 'An Incremental Approach to Self-directed Learning' *Journal of Nursing Education, 20 (6),* 30-35
Cormier, W. and Cormier, L.S. (1979) *Interviewing Strategies for Helpers. A Guide to Assessment, Treatment and Evaluation.* Brooks/Cole Pub. Co., Monterey
Coulthard, M. (1984) 'Conversation Analysis and Social Skills Training' in P. Trower (ed) *Radical Approaches to Social Skills Training.* Croom Helm, Beckenham
Cozby, P. (1973) 'Self-disclosure: A Literature Review'. *Psychological Bulletin,* 79, 73-91
Crossman, E.R. (1960) 'Automation and Skill' *D.S.I.R. Problems of Progress in Industry. No. 9,* H.M.S.O., London
Curran, J., Farrell, A. and Grunberger, A. (1984) 'Social Skills Training: A Critique and a Rapprochement' in P. Trower (ed) *Radical Approaches to Social Skills Training.* Croom Helm, Beckenham
Derlega, V. and Chaikin, A. (1975) *Sharing Intimacy: What We Reveal to Others and Why.* Prentice-Hall, New Jersey
DHSS (1972) *Report of the Committee on Nursing* (Briggs Report) H.M.S.O., London
DHSS (1975) *Better Services for the Mentally Ill.* H.M.S.O., London
Dickinson, S. (1982) 'The Nursing Process and the Professional Status of Nursing'. *Nursing Times, 78,* 16; 61-64
Eicher, J. and Kelley, E. (1972) 'High School as a Meeting Place'. *Michigan Journal of Secondary Education, 13,* 12-16
Eisler, R.M. and Frederiksen, L.W. (1980) *Perfecting Social Skills. A Guide to Interpersonal Behaviour Development.* Plenum Press, New York
Ekman, P. and Friesen, W. (1982) 'Measuring Facial Movement with the Facial Action Coding System' in P. Ekman (ed) *Emotion in the Human Face,* 2nd edn. Cambridge University Press, Cambridge
Ellis, R. and Whittington, D. (1981) *A Guide to Social Skill Training.* Croom Helm, Beckenham, Kent
Faulkner, A. (1985) 'The Evaluation of Teaching Interpersonal Skills to Nurses' in C. Kagan (ed) *Interpersonal Skills in Nursing.* Croom Helm, London
Fensterheim, H. (1972) 'Behaviour Therapy: Assertive Training in Groups' in C.J. Sager and M.S. Kaplan (eds) *Progress in Group and Family Therapy.* Brunner and Mazel, New York

Ferguson, R. and Carney, M. (1970) 'Interpersonal Considerations and Judgements in a Day Hospital'. *British Journal of Psychiatry, 117,* 397-403

Ferster, C.B. and Skinner, B.F. (1957) *Schedules of Reinforcement.* Century Crofts, New York

Field, G. and Test, M. (1975) 'Group Assertive Training for Severely Disturbed Patients'. *Journal of Behaviour Therapy and Experimental Psychiatry, 6,* 129-134

Foucault, M. (1979) *Madness and Civilization. A History of Insanity in the Age of Reason.* Tavistock Publication Co., London

Foy, D.W., Eisler, R.M. and Pinkston, S. (1975) 'Modelled Assertion in a Case of Explosive Rages'. *Journal of Behaviour Therapy and Experimental Psychiatry, 6,* 135-137

French, P. (1983) *Social Skills for Nursing Practice.* Croom Helm, London

Fry, L. (1983) 'Women in Society' in S. Spence and G. Shepherd (eds), *Developments in Social Skills Training.* Academic Press, London

Furnham, A. (1983) 'Situational Determinants of Social Skill' in R. Ellis and D. Whittington (eds) *New Directions in Social Skill Training.* Croom Helm, Beckenham, Kent

Gergen, K. and Gergen, M. (1981) *Social Psychology.* Harcourt Brace Jovanovich, New York

Goldberg, E.K. (1971) 'Effects of Models and Instructions on a Verbal Interviewing Behaviour: An Analysis of Two Factors of the Microcounselling Paradigm'. *Dissertation Abstracts International, August 737A*

Goldsmith, J. and McFall, R. (1975) 'Development and Evaluation of an Interpersonal Skill Training Program for Psychiatric Inpatients'. *Journal of Abnormal Psychology, 84,* 51-58

Greenspoon, J. (1955) 'The Reinforcing Effect of Two Spoken Sounds on the Frequency of Two Responses'. *American Journal of Psychiatry, 68,* 609-16

Gulley, H. (1968) *Discussion, Conference and Group Process,* 2nd edn, Holt, Rinehart and Winston, New York

Gustafson, M.B. (1977) 'Let's Broaden Our Horizons About the Use of Contracts'. *International Nursing Review, 24 (1),* 18-19

Gutride, M., Goldstein, A. and Hunter, G. (1973) 'The Use of Modelling and Role-playing to Increase Social Interaction Among Asocial Psychiatric Patients'. *Journal of Consulting and Clinical Psychology, 400,* 400-415

Halpern, H.M. and Lesser, L.N. (1960) 'Empathy in Infants, Adults and Psychotherapists.' *Psychoanalytical Review, 47,* 38

Hargie, O. (1986) 'Communication as Skilled Behaviour' in O. Hargie (ed) *A Handbook of Communication Skills.* Croom Helm, Beckenham, Kent

——, Saunders, C. and Dickson, D. (1981) *Social Skills in Interpersonal Communication.* Croom Helm, London

Haviland, J. and Malatesta, C. (1981) 'The Development of Sex Differences in Nonverbal Signals: Fallacies, Facts and Fantasies' in C. Mayo and N. Henley (eds) *Gender and Nonverbal Behaviour.* Springer-Verlag, New York

Heilveil, T. (1983) *Video in Mental Health Practice.* Springer, New York

Horan, J.J. (1979) *Counselling for Effective Decision Making.* Duxbury Press, Massachusetts

Insko, C. (1965) 'Verbal Reinforcement of Altitude', *Journal of Personality and Social Psychology, 2,* 261-263

Ivey, A.E. and Authier, J. (1978) *Microcounselling. Innovations in Interviewing, Counselling, Psychotherapy and Psychoeducation,* 2nd edn. Charles C. Thomas, Springfield

Ivey, A.E., Normington, C.J., Millar, C.D., Morrill, W.H. and Haase, R.F. (1968) 'Microcounselling and Attending Behaviour'. *Journal of Counselling Psychology, 15,* 1-12

Izard, E. (1977) *Human Emotions.* Plenum, New York
Jones, M. (1968) *Social Psychiatry in Practice. The Idea of the Therapeutic Community.* Penguin, Harmondsworth
Jourard, S. (1966) 'An Exploratory Study of Body-accessibility' *British Journal of Social and Clinical Psychology, 5,* 221-231
Kalisch, B. (1973) 'What is Empathy?' *American Journal of Nursing, 73* (September), 1548-1552
Keisler, S. (1978) *Interpersonal Processes in Groups and Organizations.* AHM Publishers, Arlington Heights, Illinois
Kelly, J. (1982) *Social Skills Training: A Practical Guide for Interventions.* Springer, New York
Lange, A. and Jakubowski, P. (1976) *Responsible Assertive Behaviour.* Research Press. Champaign, Illinois
Langford, T. (1972) 'Self-directed Learning'. *Nursing Outlook, 20,* 648-651
Lazarus, A. (1971) *Behaviour Therapy and Beyond.* McGraw-Hill, New York
Leeper, R. (1935) 'The Role of Motivation in Learning: A Study of the Phenomenon of Different Motivation Control of the Utilisation of Habits'. *Journal of Genetic Psychology, 46,* 3-40
Liberman, R., King, L., De Risi, W. and McCann, M. (1975) *Personal Effectiveness.* Research Press. Champaign, Illinois
Libet, J.M. and Lewinsohn, P.M. (1973) 'Concept of Social Skill with Special References to the Behaviour of Depressed Patients'. *Journal of Consulting and Clinical Psychology, 40,* 304-312
Linehan, M. and Egan, K. (1979) 'Assertion Training for Women' in A. Bellack and M. Hersen (eds) *Research and Practice in Social Skills Training.* Plenum, New York
Longabaugh, R., Eldred, S.H., Bell, N.W. and Sherman, L.J. (1966) 'The International World of the Chronic Schizophrenic Patient'. *Psychiatry, 29,* 319-44
Loomis, M. (1985) 'Levels of Contracting'. *Journal of Psychosocial Nursing and Mental Health Services,* March, *Vol. 23,* No. 3
Luft, J. (1969) *On Human Interaction.* National Press, Palo Alto, California
Magnusson, D. (1981) *Towards a Psychology of Situations.* Lawrence Erlbaum, Hillsdale, New Jersey
Maloney, E. (1962) Does the Psychiatric Nurse have Independent Functions?' *American Journal of Nursing 62,* 61-3, June 62
Marks, I.M., Connoly, J., Hallam, R. and Philpott, R. (1975) 'Nurse Therapists in Behavioural Psychotherapy'. *British Medical Journal, iii,* 144-148
Marshall, W.L. and McKnight, R.D. (1975) 'An Integrated Program for Sexual Offenders'. *Canadian Psychiatric Association Journal, 20,* 133-138
Martin, D.V. (1974) *Adventure in Psychiatry,* 2nd edn. Bruno Cassirer, Oxford
Marzillier, J.A., Lambert, C. and Kellett, J. (1976) 'A Controlled Evaluation of Systematic Desensitization and Social Skills Training for Socially Inadequate Psychiatric Patients'. *Behaviour Research and Therapy, 14,* 225-238
Marzillier, J.S. and Winter, K. (1978) 'Success and Failure in Social Skills Training: Individual Differences'. *Behaviour Research and Therapy, 16,* 67-84
Maslow, A. (1954) *Motivation and Personality.* Harper and Row, New York
Mayo, C. and Henley, N. (1981) 'Nonverbal Behaviour: Barrier or Agent for Sex Role Change' in C. Mayo and N. Henley (eds) *Gender and Nonverbal Behaviour.* Springer-Verlag, New York
McFall, A. (1982) 'A Review and Reformulation of the Concept of Social Skills'. *Behavioural Assessment, 4,* 1-33
Milroy, E. (1982) *Role-play: A Practical Guide.* Aberdeen University Press, Aberdeen
Ministry of Health Central Services Council (1968) *Psychiatric Nursing: Today*

and Tomorrow, H.M.S.O., London

Monti, P., Corriveau, D. and Curran, J. (1982) 'Social Skills Training for Psychiatric Patients: Treatment and Outcome' in J. Curran and P. Monti (eds) *Social Skills Training: A Practical Handbook for Assessment and Treatment.* Guilford Press, New York

Moore, M.F., Barber, J.H., Robinson, E.T. and Taylore, T.R. (1973) 'First Contact Decisions in General Practice'. *Lancet, i,* 817-819

Morris, D. (1971) *Intimate Behaviour.* Cape, London

Napier, R. and Gershenfeld, M. (1973) *Groups: Theory and Experience.* Houghton Mifflin, Boston

National Board for Nursing, Midwifery & Health Visiting (1983) Syllabus for Part 3 of the Register of Nurses, Midwives and Health Visitors. Mental Nursing

Neisser, U. (1967) *Cognitive Psychology.* Appleton-Century-Crofts, New York

Nelson-Jones, R. (1982) *The Theory and Practice of Counselling Psychology.* Holt, Rinehart and Winston, London

Oei, T.P.S. and Jackson, P. (1980) 'Long-term Effects of Group and Individual Social Skills Training with Alcoholics'. *Addictive Behaviours, 5,* 129-136

O'Hare, B. (1972) 'Working with Small Groups' (Foreword: Part 1) *Nursing Times, 68,* 153

O'Leary, D.E., O'Leary, M.R. and Donovan, D.M. (1976) 'Social Skill Acquisition and Psychological Development of Alcoholics: A Review.' *Addictive Behaviours, 1,* 111-120

Panepinto, R.A. (1976) 'Social Skills Training for Verbally Aggressive Children'. *Unpublished doctoral dissertation.* University of West Virginia

Peck, D. (1973) 'The Psychiatric Nurse as Therapist 1. An Agent of Behaviour Change.' *Nursing Times, 69 (35),* 139

Phillips, E.L. (1985) 'Social Skills: History and Prospect' in L. L'Abate and M. Milan (eds). *Handbook of Social Skills Training and Research.* Wiley, New York

Pillay, M. and Crisp, A.H. (1977) 'The Impact of SST Within an Established In-patient Treatment Programme for Anorexia Nervosa.' *British Journal of Psychiatry, 39,* 533-539

Priestley, P. and McGuire, J. (1983) *Learning to Help. Basic Skills Exercises.* Tavistock Publications, London

——, ——, Flegg, D., Hemsley, V. and Welham, D. (1978) *Social Skills and Personal Problem Solving.* Tavistock Publications, London

Rakos, R. (1986) 'Asserting and Confronting' in O. Hargie (ed) *A Handbook of Communication Skills.* Croom Helm, Beckenham, Kent

Rice, E.M. and Chaplin, T.C. (1979) 'Social Skills Training for Hospitalized Male Arsonists'. *Journal of Behavioural Therapy and Experimental Psychiatry, 10,* 105-108

Rosenfeld, H.M. and Hancks, M. (1980) 'The Nonverbal Context of Verbal Listener Responses' in M.R. Key (ed) *The Relationship of Verbal and Nonverbal Communication,* Mouton, The Hague

Rosenshine, B. (1971) *Teaching Behaviours and Student Achievement.* NFER-Nelson Publishing Co., London

Roth, H.L. (1889) 'On Salutations' *Journal of the Royal Anthropological Institute, 19,* 164-181

Roth, I. (1976) *Social Perception.* Open University Press, Milton Keynes

Royal College of Psychiatrists (1973) The Future of Psychiatric Services in Scotland (Tait Report). Edinburgh

Russell, G.F.M. (1973) 'Will There be Enough Psychiatrists to Run a Psychiatric Service Based on District General Hospitals?' in R. Cawley and G. McLachlan (eds). *Policy for Action.* Oxford University Press, London

Rutter, M. (1972) *Maternal Deprivation Reassessed.* Penguin, Harmondsworth

Sabshin, M. (1957) 'Nurse-Doctor-Patient Relationships in Psychiatry'. *American Journal of Nursing, 57 (2)* 188-192

Sarason, T.G. and Ganzer, V.S. (1973) 'Modelling and Group Discussion in the Rehabilitation of Juvenile Delinquents.' *Journal of Counselling Psychology, 20,* 442-449

Schafer, R. (1959) Generative Empathy in the Treatment Situation. *Psychoanalytical Quarterly, 28,* 345

Scherer, K., Fortin, F., Spitzer, W.O. and Kergin, D.J. (1977) 'Nurse-Practitioners in Primary Care (VII): A Cohort Study of 99 Nurses and 79 Associated Physicians'. *Canadian Medical Association Journal, 116,* 856-862

—— and Ekman, P. (1982) (eds). *Handbook of Methods in Nonverbal Behaviour Research.* Cambridge University Press, Cambridge

Shapiro, J.G. (1968) 'Responsivity to Facial and Linguistic Cues'. *Journal of Communication, 18,* 11-17

Shaw, B. (1979) 'The Theoretical and Experimental Foundations of a Cognitive Model for Depression' in P. Pliner, K. Blankstein and I. Spigel (eds) *Advances in the Study of Communication: Volume 5.* Plenum, New York

Shaw, M. (1981) *Group Dynamics. The Psychology of Small Group Behaviour,* 3rd edn. McGraw-Hill, New York

Shepherd, G. and Spence, S. (1983) 'Concluding Comments' in S. Spence and G. Shepherd (eds). *Developments in Social Skills Training.* Academic Press, London

Skinner, B.F. (1953) *Science and Human Behaviour.* Collier MacMillan, London

Smith, V. (1986) 'Listening' in O. Hargie (ed) *A Handbook of Communication Skills,* Croom Helm, Beckenham, Kent

Spence, S. (1980) *Social Skills Training with Children and Adolescents.* NFER, Windsor

Stewart, R., Powell, G. and Chetwynd, S. (1979) *Person Perception and Stereotyping.* Saxon House, Farnborough, England

Stonehill, E. and Crisp, A.H. (1977) 'Psychoneurotic Characteristics of Patients with Anorexia Nervosa Before and After Treatment and at Follow-up 4-7 Years Later.' *Journal of Psychosomatic Research, 21,* 187-193

Stuart, G.W. and Sundeen, S.J. (1983) *Principles and Practice of Psychiatric Nursing,* 2nd edn. The C.V. Mosby Company, St Louis

Travelbee, J. (1971) *Interpersonal Aspects of Nursing,* 2nd edn. F.A. Davis Co., Philadelphia

Trick, K.L.K. and Obcarskas, C. (1968) *Understanding Mental Illness and Its Nursing,* 1st edn., Pitman Medical Publishing Co Ltd., London

Trower, P., Bryant, B. and Argyle, M. (1978) *Social Skills and Mental Health.* Methuen, London

Turney, C., Cairns, L., Williams, G., Hatton, N. and Owens, L. (1973) *Sydney Micro Skills: Series 1 Handbook.* Sydney University Press, Sydney, Australia

Turney, C., Owens, L., Hatton, N., Williams, G. and Cairns, L. (1976) *Sydney Micro Skills: Series 2 Handbook.* Sydney University Press, Sydney, Australia

Ullrich de Muynck, R. and Ullrich, R. (1972) 'The Efficiency of a Standardised Assertive Training Program'. *Paper presented at Second Conference of European Association for Behaviour Therapy and Modification.* Wexford, Ireland

United Kingdom Central Council for Nursing, Midwifery and Health Visiting (1982) *Education and Training.* Consultation Paper 1

Van den Pol, R., Iwata, B.A., Ivanck, M.T., Page, T.J., Neef, N.A. and Whitley, F.P. (1981) 'Teaching the Handicapped to Eat in Public Places'. *Journal of Applied Behavioural Analysis, 14,* 61-69

Van Hasselt, V., Hersen, M. and Milliones, J. (1978) 'Social Skills Training for Alcoholics and Drug Addicts: A Review'. *Addictive Behaviour, 3,* 221-233

——, ——, Whitehill, M. and Bellack, A. (1979) 'Social Skill Assessment and Training for Children: An Evaluative Review'. *Behaviour Research and Therapy, 17,* 413-437

Warr, P. and Knapper, C. (1968) *The Perception of People and Events.* Wiley, London

Welford, A. (1958) *Ageing and Human Skill.* Oxford University Press, London. Reprinted 1973 by Greenwood Press, Connecticut

—— (1965) 'Performance, Biological Mechanisms and Age: A Theoretical Sketch' in A. Welford and J. Birren (eds). *Behaviour, Ageing and the Nervous System.* C.C. Thomas, Illinois

—— (1980) 'The Concept of Skill and Its Application to Social Performance' in W. Singleton, P. Spurgeon and R. Stammers (eds). *The Analysis of Social Skill.* Plenum, New York

Wells, K.C., Hersen, M., Bellack, A.S. and Himmelhock, M.D. (1979) 'SST in Unipolar Nonpsychotic Depression'. *American Journal of Psychology, 136,* 1331-1332

Wessler, R. (1984) 'Cognitive-Social Psychological Theories and Social Skills: A Review' in P. Trower (ed) *Radical Approaches to Social Skills Training* Croom Helm, Beckenham, Kent

Westland, G. (1980) 'Social Skills Training with Epileptic Psychiatric Patients.' *Occupational Therapy, Jan.,* pp. 13-16

Whitehead, J.A. and Fannon, D. (1971) 'A Clinical Role for Senior Nurses.' *Lancet, ii,* 756-758

Wilkinson, J. and Canter, S. (1983) *Social Skills Training Manual. Assessment, Programme Design and Management of Training.* John Wiley & Sons, Chichester

Wing, J.K. and Brown, G.W. (1970) *Institutionalism and Schizophrenia.* Cambridge University Press, Cambridge

Wolpe, J. (1958) *Psychotherapy by Reciprocal Inhibition.* Stanford University Press, California

AUTHOR INDEX

Alberti, R. 179, 187, 230
Altschul, A. 38
Annett, J. 57
Argyle, M. 3, 12, 17, 21, 41, 42, 43, 65
Arvey, R. 60
Athos, A. 209, 212
Authier, J. 120, 209, 210
Averill, J. 52

Bandura, A. 6, 10, 31, 55
Barton, R. 14
Beckmann-Murray 207
Becvar, R. 209
Bernstein, B. 56
Bird, J. 37
Birdwhistell, R. 126
Blondis, M. 200
Brammer, L. 201
Briggs, K. 108
Brown, G. 14
Bruner, J. 63
Bryant, B. 12
Bull, P. 128
Butler, R. 28

Campion, J. 60
Canter, S. 104
Carney, M. 38
Centres, R. 219
Chaikin, A. 146
Chaplin, T. 21
Christoff, K. 245
Cook, M. 59, 61, 69
Coombe, E. 115
Cormier, L. 210, 213
Cormier, W. 210, 213
Coulthard, W. 210, 213
Cozby, P. 152
Crisp, A. 21
Crossman, E. 23
Curran, J. 51

Derlega, V. 46
Dickinson, S. 36

Egan, K. 183

Eicher, J. 70
Eisler, R. 107, 115
Ekman, P. 54, 138
Ellis, R. 1
Emmons, M. 179, 187, 230

Fannon, D. 38
Faulkner, A. 111
Fensterheim, H. 21
Ferguson, R. 38
Ferster, C. 217
Field, G. 23
Fouchault, M. 33
Foy, D. 21
Frederiksen, L. 107, 115
French, P. 206, 209
Friesen, W. 138
Fry, L. 186
Furnham, A. 68

Gabarro, J. 209, 212
Ganzer, V. 22
Gergen, K. 71, 189
Gergen, M. 71, 189
Gershenfeld, M. 190
Goldberg, E. 214
Goldsmith, J. 23
Greenspoon, J. 219
Gulley, H. 192
Gustafson, M. 115
Gutridge, M. 22

Halpern, H. 208
Hancks, M. 197
Hargie, O. 2, 4, 164, 196, 199, 209, 210, 212, 213
Haviland, J. 68
Heilveil, T. 96
Henley, N. 68
Horan, J. 209

Insko, C. 219
Ivey, A. 120, 209, 210, 214
Izard, E. 51

Jackson, B. 200
Jackson, P. 22

253

SUBJECT INDEX

For Product Safety Concerns and Information please contact our EU representative GPSR@taylorandfrancis.com
Taylor & Francis Verlag GmbH, Kaufingerstraße 24, 80331 München, Germany